Mycoplasma bovis Infections

Mycoplasma bovis Infections: Occurrence, Pathogenesis, Diagnosis and Control, Including Prevention and Therapy

Editors

Katarzyna Dudek
Ewelina Szacawa

MDPI • Basel • Beijing • Wuhan • Barcelona • Belgrade • Manchester • Tokyo • Cluj • Tianjin

Editors
Katarzyna Dudek
National Veterinary Research Institute
Poland

Ewelina Szacawa
National Veterinary Research Institute
Poland

Editorial Office
MDPI
St. Alban-Anlage 66
4052 Basel, Switzerland

This is a reprint of articles from the Special Issue published online in the open access journal *Pathogens* (ISSN 2076-0817) (available at: https://www.mdpi.com/journal/pathogens/special_issues/mycoplasma_bovis_infections).

For citation purposes, cite each article independently as indicated on the article page online and as indicated below:

LastName, A.A.; LastName, B.B.; LastName, C.C. Article Title. *Journal Name* **Year**, *Volume Number*, Page Range.

ISBN 978-3-0365-0194-9 (Hbk)
ISBN 978-3-0365-0195-6 (PDF)

Contents

About the Editors vii

Katarzyna Dudek and Ewelina Szacawa
Mycoplasma bovis Infections: Occurrence, Pathogenesis, Diagnosis and Control, Including Prevention and Therapy
Reprinted from: *Pathogens* **2020**, *9*, 994, doi:10.3390/pathogens9120994 . . . . **1**

Katarzyna Dudek, Robin A. J. Nicholas, Ewelina Szacawa and Dariusz Bednarek
Mycoplasma bovis Infections—Occurrence, Diagnosis and Control
Reprinted from: *Pathogens* **2020**, *9*, 640, doi:10.3390/pathogens9080640 . . . . **5**

Katarzyna Dudek, Dariusz Bednarek, Urszula Lisiecka, Anna Kycko, Michał Reichert, Krzysztof Kostro and Stanisław Winiarczyk
Analysis of the Leukocyte Response in Calves Suffered from *Mycoplasma bovis* Pneumonia
Reprinted from: *Pathogens* **2020**, *9*, 407, doi:10.3390/pathogens9050407 . . . . **27**

Mette Bisgaard Petersen, Lars Pedersen, Lone Møller Pedersen and Liza Rosenbaum Nielsen
Field Experience of Antibody Testing against *Mycoplasma bovis* in Adult Cows in Commercial Danish Dairy Cattle Herds
Reprinted from: *Pathogens* **2020**, *9*, 637, doi:10.3390/pathogens9080637 . . . . **39**

Salvatore Catania, Michele Gastaldelli, Eliana Schiavon, Andrea Matucci, Annalucia Tondo, Marianna Merenda and Robin A. J. Nicholas
Infection Dynamics of *Mycoplasma bovis* and Other Respiratory Mycoplasmas in Newly Imported Bulls on Italian Fattening Farms
Reprinted from: *Pathogens* **2020**, *9*, 537, doi:10.3390/pathogens9070537 . . . . **55**

Tarja Pohjanvirta, Nella Vähänikkilä, Henri Simonen, Sinikka Pelkonen and Tiina Autio
Efficacy of Two Antibiotic-Extender Combinations on *Mycoplasma bovis* in Bovine Semen Production
Reprinted from: *Pathogens* **2020**, *9*, 808, doi:10.3390/pathogens9100808 . . . . **65**

Lisa Ledger, Jason Eidt and Hugh Yuehua Cai
Identification of Antimicrobial Resistance-Associated Genes through Whole Genome Sequencing of *Mycoplasma bovis* Isolates with Different Antimicrobial Resistances
Reprinted from: *Pathogens* **2020**, *9*, 588, doi:10.3390/pathogens9070588 . . . . **77**

Andrea Kinnear, Tim A. McAllister, Rahat Zaheer, Matthew Waldner, Antonio C. Ruzzini, Sara Andrés-Lasheras, Sarah Parker, Janet E. Hill and Murray D. Jelinski
Investigation of Macrolide Resistance Genotypes in *Mycoplasma bovis* Isolates from Canadian Feedlot Cattle
Reprinted from: *Pathogens* **2020**, *9*, 622, doi:10.3390/pathogens9080622 . . . . **91**

Claire A.M. Becker, Chloé Ambroset, Anthéa Huleux, Angélique Vialatte, Adélie Colin, Agnès Tricot, Marie-Anne Arcangioli and Florence Tardy
Monitoring *Mycoplasma bovis* Diversity and Antimicrobial Susceptibility in Calf Feedlots Undergoing a Respiratory Disease Outbreak
Reprinted from: *Pathogens* **2020**, *9*, 593, doi:10.3390/pathogens9070593 . . . . **107**

About the Editors

Katarzyna Dudek graduated in Veterinary Medicine at the University of Life Sciences in Lublin (Poland) and received a PhD in Animal Physiology from the same institution. In 2019, she received a DSc degree in Agricultural Sciences in the discipline of Veterinary Sciences from the National Veterinary Research Institute in Pulawy (Poland) where she has been working since 2006. Her main activities and responsibilities involve diagnostics of ruminant mycoplasmas, veterinary immunology, and Mycoplasma bovis vaccine studies. She is the author of 49 review and research papers featured in the Journal and Citation Reports list.

Ewelina Szacawa graduated in Biotechnology at the University of Life Sciences in Lublin (Poland). Since 2008, she has been working in the National Veterinary Research Institute in Pulawy (Poland) where she obtained her PhD in Veterinary Sciences in 2016. Her main researches are focused on diagnostics of ruminant mycoplasmas, veterinary immunology, and molecular studies on Mycoplasma bovis. She has published 15 papers listed in Journal and Citation Reports.

pathogens

MDPI

Editorial

Mycoplasma bovis Infections: Occurrence, Pathogenesis, Diagnosis and Control, Including Prevention and Therapy

Katarzyna Dudek * and Ewelina Szacawa

Department of Cattle and Sheep Diseases, National Veterinary Research Institute, 57 Partyzantów Avenue, 24100 Pulawy, Poland; ewelina.szacawa@piwet.pulawy.pl

* Correspondence: katarzyna.dudek@piwet.pulawy.pl

Received: 23 November 2020; Accepted: 23 November 2020; Published: 27 November 2020

Mycoplasma bovis (*M. bovis*) is an etiological agent of bronchopneumonia, mastitis, arthritis, otitis, keratoconjunctivitis, meningitis, endocarditis and other disorders in cattle. It is known to spread worldwide, including countries for a long time considered free of the infection. This editorial summarizes the data described in the Special Issue entitled "*Mycoplasma bovis* Infections: Occurrence, Pathogenesis, Diagnosis and Control, Including Prevention and Therapy" consisting of eight research articles and a review. The research articles discuss the most important issues related to *Mycoplasma bovis* infections, including the lung local immunity in *M. bovis* pneumonia, antimicrobial susceptibility and antimicrobial resistance-associated genes of *M. bovis* isolates, *M. bovis* antibody testing, efficacy of seminal extender on *M. bovis* as well as imported bull examination for *M. bovis*, whereas the latest data were summarized in the review.

The review of this Issue summarized the latest data on *Mycoplasma bovis* infections, introducing the problem, taking into account the issues related to spread of *M. bovis* around the world, the disease therapy and immunoprophylaxis of the infections. It discussed the current epizootic situation of *M. bovis*, including the studies from the countries for a long time considered free of *M. bovis*, such as Finland, New Zealand or Australia. The review listed the most important courses of *M. bovis* infection and their sources including colostrum, milk, air-borne, intrauterine and newly noticed semen. An important part of the review was also devoted to the description of currently used methods in the diagnosis of *M. bovis*, especially in terms of the specimen used. The review also addressed the issue of methods of the disease eradication and collected the most important recommendations in order to unify the rules of preventing *M. bovis* infections in the designed control programs [1].

The research article by Dudek et al. [2] described the leukocyte response in *M. bovis* pneumonia using the calf infection model. In the experimentally infected calves, the lung immune response manifested in both the T- and B-lymphocyte stimulation. The local immunity was also characterized by the increased phagocyte expression and upregulation of antigen-presenting mechanisms dependent on the MHC class II. On the other hand, the activation of peripheral antimicrobial mechanisms was manifested in the general stimulation of phagocytic activity and oxygen metabolism of leukocytes, however it depended on the stage of the disease.

The work of Petersen et al. [3] aimed to compare two commercially available ELISAs for *M. bovis* antibody detection in adult cows from 12 dairy herds with a known previous *M. bovis* infection status. With the use of the newly commercially released ELISA, more positive serum and milk samples were diagnosed compared to the second of the tested tests, which proved its higher sensitivity. Additional analysis of the concordance correlation coefficient of sample-to-positive percentage showed high comparability between the serum and milk samples for this test; however, with the higher serum values. These results indicate that the milk samples are a good matrix for *M. bovis* antibody testing in this test as the serum samples and can be used as a replacer. As a result of this study, the suitability of the newly commercially released ELISA for the evaluation of subclinically infected animals and bull tank milk samples as well as for herd-level control was proposed. However, the specificity of this test was questioned, which may be related to cross-reactions presence. In the authors' opinion, the second of the tested tests seems to be useful primarily for detection of clinically ill animals.

The research article by Catania et al. [4] discussed the role of newly imported bulls in spreading of bovine mycoplasmas in fattening farms, including *M. bovis*. In 19.1% of total of 711 nasal swabs three times collected (on arrival, at 15 and 60 days after arrival), *M. bovis* was isolated as poor or mixed cultures with other species of the *Mollicutes* class. The results showed a clear dependence of *M. bovis* prevalence on the sampling time. On arrival, the majority of bulls tested were free of *M. bovis*. Significantly increased *M. bovis* prevalence was observed 15 days after arrival which ranged between 40 and 81% dependent on the method used, whereas general its decrease was noted 45 days after. Here, there was also no predictive role of environmental conditions in *M. bovis* prevalence in the imported bulls.

The study of Pohjanvirta et al. [5] drew attention to the real risk of *M. bovis* transmission via artificial insemination in the context of the poor mycoplasmacidal efficacy of antibiotics used in the semen extender. The efficacy of the combinations of antibiotics added to the semen extender used in this study was dependent on the *M. bovis* concentration in spiked semen samples and differed in the case of the two tested bacterial strains, ATCC and wild type. Additionally, from all three tested DNA extraction methods, the one with the highest sensitivity for detection of either of the *M. bovis* strains in the pools spiked with low concentration of the pathogen was selected. To prevent the transmission of *M. bovis* via the contaminated semen, the authors suggested using a higher than recommended combination of antibiotics added to the semen extender, or which would be the best solution to test bulls intended for artificial insemination for *M. bovis* and use semen free of the pathogen.

Ledger et al. [6] covered the topic in the field of increasing resistance of *M. bovis* isolates for antimicrobials that was reported in many countries. This article describes the antimicrobial resistance-associated genes in *M. bovis* isolate from 2019 that had high minimum inhibitory concentration (MIC) for fluorochinolones, tetracyclines, macrolides, lincosamides and pleuromutulins. With the use of whole genome sequencing (WGS) more non-synonymous mutations and gene disruptions were identified in the recently received *M. bovis* isolate when compared with the past isolate and reference strain PG45. The researchers selected 55 genes for the potential function of antimicrobial resistance. It gives the possibility to further analyze this candidate AMR genes and compare it with another research in the future.

The main aim of the work of Kinnear et al. [7] was to assess the relationship between the genotypes and phenotypes of *M. bovis* isolates in the evaluation of antimicrobial resistance to macrolides, used both in the prevention and treatment of *M. bovis* infections in feedlot cattle. In this cross-sectional twelve-year study a total of 126 *M. bovis* isolates were tested. The samples originated from feedlot cattle of different health status and were collected from multiple anatomical locations. The MIC values for five selected macrolides were estimated following the antimicrobial susceptibility testing. Additionally, the genotype of all isolates based on the number and positions of single nucleotide polymorphisms (mutations) in the 23S rRNA gene alleles and ribosomal proteins was determined. The efficacy of the examined macrolides was depended on the type of mutations determined for each *M. bovis* isolate, with exception of tildipirosin and tilmicosin, which, according to the authors, seem to be unsuitable for *M. bovis* infection treatment in cattle.

The two-year study of Becker et al. [8] concerned longitudinal monitoring of *M. bovis* infections in 25 feedlots. It revealed that the low *M. bovis* prevalence was observed in calves at their arrival in the feedlot, whereas the high prevalence was seen 4 weeks after the antimicrobial treatment. This at indicates the ineffective antimicrobial treatment of the infected calves due to antibiotic resistance of *M. bovis* strains. The important finding was that these strains were resistant to antibiotics prior to any treatments of the calves and it led to the clinical recovery of animals without *M. bovis* clearance. This research supports the previous finding about the overall multiresistance of *M. bovis* isolates to the most of the tested antimicrobials except for fluoroquinolones and that the most strains belonged to little variable subtype ST2, based on the single-locus sequence analysis of *polC* gene.

García-Galán et al. [9] described the research on *M. bovis* isolated from beef and dairy cattle. According to the study, this pathogen was present in 40.9% of examined beef cattle and in 16.36% of dairy cattle. The MIC testing and WGS results showed that the most isolates were resistant to many antimicrobials (macrolides, lincosamides and tetracyclines). The genome sequencing also revealed that the *M. bovis* isolates belonged to only two STs (ST2 and ST3). The research revealed that the most isolates that belonged to ST3 had high MIC values for fluoroquinolones and the ST2 isolates had lower MIC values for this group of antimicrobials. The researchers also showed that the main differences between the ST2 and ST3 were located in the quinolone-resistance determining regions of *GyrA* and *ParC* genes. The mutations in these genes were found only in the *M. bovis* isolates belonged to ST3. In vitro testing revealed that only valnemulin was effective against the *M. bovis* isolates from both STs.

The articles included in this Special Issue present the most up-to-date data on *M. bovis* infections, including the disease pathogenesis and therapy, and contribute significantly to improving knowledge in this field.

Author Contributions: Conceptualization, K.D.; Writing—Original draft preparation, K.D., E.S.; Writing—Review and Editing, K.D., E.S. All authors have read and agreed to the published version of the manuscript.

Funding: This research received no external funding.

Acknowledgments: We would like to thank all the authors of the nine papers published in this Special Issue.

Conflicts of Interest: The authors declare no conflict of interest.

References

1. Dudek, K.; Nicholas, R.A.J.; Szacawa, E.; Bednarek, D. *Mycoplasma bovis* Infections—Occurrence, Diagnosis and Control. *Pathogens* **2020**, *9*, 640. [CrossRef] [PubMed]
2. Dudek, K.; Bednarek, D.; Lisiecka, U.; Kycko, A.; Reichert, M.; Kostro, K.; Winiarczyk, S. Analysis of the Leukocyte Response in Calves Suffered from *Mycoplasma bovis* Pneumonia. *Pathogens* **2020**, *9*, 407. [CrossRef] [PubMed]
3. Petersen, M.B.; Pedersen, L.; Pedersen, L.M.; Nielsen, L.R. Field Experience of Antibody Testing against *Mycoplasma bovis* in Adult Cows in Commercial Danish Dairy Cattle Herds. *Pathogens* **2020**, *9*, 637. [CrossRef] [PubMed]
4. Catania, S.; Gastaldelli, M.; Schiavon, E.; Matucci, A.; Tondo, A.; Merenda, M.; Nicholas, R.A.J. Infection Dynamics of *Mycoplasma bovis* and Other Respiratory Mycoplasmas in Newly Imported Bulls on Italian Fattening Farms. *Pathogens* **2020**, *9*, 537. [CrossRef] [PubMed]
5. Pohjanvirta, T.; Vähänikkilä, N.; Simonen, H.; Pelkonen, S.; Autio, T. Efficacy of Two Antibiotic-Extender Combinations on *Mycoplasma bovis* in Bovine Semen Production. *Pathogens* **2020**, *9*, 808. [CrossRef] [PubMed]
6. Ledger, L.; Eidt, J.; Cai, H.Y. Identification of Antimicrobial Resistance-Associated Genes through Whole Genome Sequencing of *Mycoplasma bovis* Isolates with Different Antimicrobial Resistances. *Pathogens* **2020**, *9*, 588. [CrossRef] [PubMed]
7. Kinnear, A.; McAllister, T.A.; Zaheer, R.; Waldner, M.; Ruzzini, A.C.; Andrés-Lasheras, S.; Parker, S.; Hill, J.E.; Jelinski, M.D. Investigation of Macrolide Resistance Genotypes in *Mycoplasma bovis* Isolates from Canadian Feedlot Cattle. *Pathogens* **2020**, *9*, 622. [CrossRef] [PubMed]
8. Becker, C.A.; Ambroset, C.; Huleux, A.; Vialatte, A.; Colin, A.; Tricot, A.; Arcangioli, M.-A.; Tardy, F. Monitoring *Mycoplasma bovis* Diversity and Antimicrobial Susceptibility in Calf Feedlots Undergoing a Respiratory Disease Outbreak. *Pathogens* **2020**, *9*, 593. [CrossRef] [PubMed]
9. García-Galán, A.; Nouvel, L.-X.; Baranowski, E.; Gómez-Martín, Á.; Sánchez, A.; Citti, C.; de la Fe, C. *Mycoplasma bovis* in Spanish Cattle Herds: Two Groups of Multiresistant Isolates Predominate, with One Remaining Susceptible to Fluoroquinolones. *Pathogens* **2020**, *9*, 545. [CrossRef] [PubMed]

pathogens

MDPI

Review

Mycoplasma bovis Infections—Occurrence, Diagnosis and Control

Katarzyna Dudek [1,*], Robin A. J. Nicholas [2], Ewelina Szacawa [1] and Dariusz Bednarek [1]

1 Department of Cattle and Sheep Diseases, National Veterinary Research Institute, 57 Partyzantów Avenue, 24100 Pulawy, Poland; ewelina.szacawa@piwet.pulawy.pl (E.S.); dbednarek@piwet.pulawy.pl (D.B.)

2 The Oaks, Nutshell Lane, Farnham, Surrey GU9 0HG, UK; robin.a.j.nicholas@gmail.com

* Correspondence: katarzyna.dudek@piwet.pulawy.pl

Received: 30 June 2020; Accepted: 4 August 2020; Published: 6 August 2020

Abstract: *Mycoplasma bovis* is a cause of bronchopneumonia, mastitis and arthritis but may also affect other main organs in cattle such us the eye, ear or brain. Despite its non-zoonotic character, *M. bovis* infections are responsible for substantial economic health and welfare problems worldwide. *M. bovis* has spread worldwide, including to countries for a long time considered free of the pathogen. Control of *M. bovis* infections is hampered by a lack of effective vaccines and treatments due to increasing trends in antimicrobial resistance. This review summarizes the latest data on the epizootic situation of *M. bovis* infections and new sources/routes of transmission of the infection, and discusses the progress in diagnostics. The review includes various recommendations and suggestions which could be applied to infection control programs.

Keywords: *Mycoplasma bovis*; cattle; disease; prevalence; control

1. Introduction

In 2017, New Zealand became the last of the major cattle-rearing countries to be infected with *Mycoplasma bovis* [1]. Finland had also remained free until relatively recently but became infected via imported cattle in 2012 [2]. Undoubtedly, *M. bovis* is now the most important mycoplasma of livestock being a primary cause of mastitis, arthritis, keratoconjunctivitis and other disorders as well as a major player in the bovine respiratory disease complex (BRD) [3]. Previously *Mycoplasma mycoides* subsp. *mycoides*, the aetiological agent of the World Organisation for Animal Health (OIE)-listed contagious bovine pleuropneumonia, had this dubious distinction but this mycoplasma is now confined to countries in sub Saharan Africa.

Mycoplasma bovis was first reported in the USA in 1961 from a case of bovine mastitis then was probably exported in cattle of high genetic quality to Israel [3]. It then spread around the world, reaching the UK and the rest of Europe in the mid1970s (Figure 1). International trade in cattle and cattle products like semen has enabled its silent spread to all continents where cattle are kept. The date of isolation in a particular country, of course, is not necessarily the date of introduction even in the USA as mycoplasmas were very much an unknown quantity and their fastidious nature made isolation and detection an extremely difficult task. Indeed, it has only been in the last two decades with the introduction of DNA amplification techniques that detection and identification have become routine in many parts of the world. However, not all countries have veterinary diagnostic laboratories which can identify these organisms.

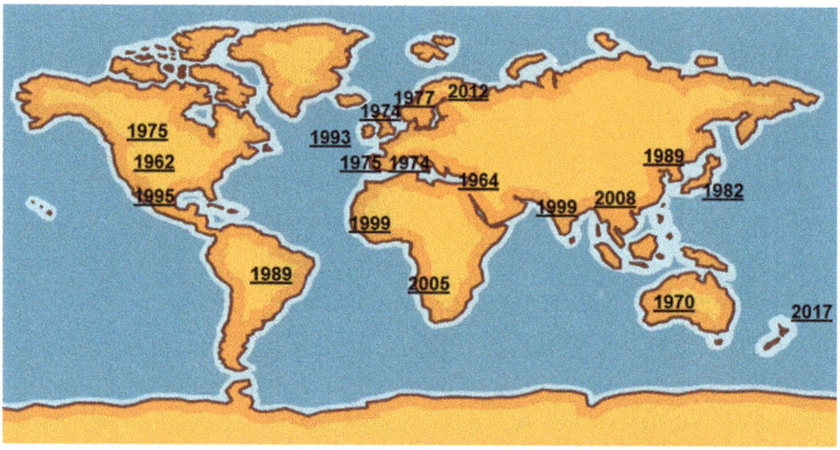

Figure 1. First detections of *Mycoplasma bovis* around the world.

Initially the importance of *M. bovis*, particularly in BRD, was underestimated because of the promotion of more established and easier detectable organisms like the bacteria *Mannheimia haemolytica*, *Histophilus somni* and *Pasteurella multocida* and viruses, namely bovine respiratory syncytial disease, parainfluenza-3 virus, bovine herpesviruses, coronaviruses and bovine viral diarrhoea virus. The presence of *M. bovis* in healthy cattle, although at a much lower levels than infected ones, delayed recognition of its pathogenicity. Once the importance of environmental factors such as weather, variation in strain virulence and its interaction with the BRD pathogens were known, studies quickly demonstrated its widespread prevalence in pneumonic calves and, later, older cattle.

Despite attempts going back nearly half a century, control of *M. bovis* diseases is still problematic because of a lack of an effective commercial vaccine. Many have been marketed, particularly in the USA, but little data exist to assess their immunogenicity and protective properties [4]. To be valuable they are required to be part of multivalent vaccines incorporating the causative bacteria and viruses currently available for BRD. Presently, no vaccine is available for mycoplasma mastitis, a major problem in large dairy herds of North America where they are often untreatable. Indeed, the major trend in the last two decades has been the alarming decrease in susceptibility of *M. bovis* to the commonly used antimicrobials including the fluoroquinolones [5].

This review summarizes the latest data on the epizootic situation of *M. bovis* infections and new sources/routes of transmission of the infection and discusses the progress in diagnostics. The review also covers aspects related to *M. bovis* infection control, collecting various recommendations and suggestions which could be applied in the infection control programs.

2. *Mycoplasma bovis*: Key Facts

Mycoplasma bovis (*M. bovis*) is most often considered to cause caseonecrotic pneumonia, mastitis and arthritis [6,7]. However, cases of infectious keratoconjunctivitis, suppurative otitis media, meningitis, decubital abscesses, endocarditis and reproductive disorders have been associated with *M. bovis* [7–10]. Most importantly *M. bovis* is one of the causes of BRD with other aetiological agents, both bacterial and viral [11,12].

M. bovis is one of 13 species of mycoplasmas diagnosed in cattle; however, not all of them cause serious diseases, and some may even constitute normal flora of the bovine respiratory tract. For example, the most important mycoplasma in bovine severe respiratory diseases is the previously mentioned *Mycoplasma mycoides* subsp. *mycoides*. *Mycoplasma bovigenitalium* is generally associated with bovine reproductive disorders, while *Mycoplasma bovoculi* has been isolated from infectious keratoconjunctivitis in cattle [3]. *M. bovis* infections are non-zoonotic; however, substantial economic and cattle health and welfare impacts are felt worldwide [3]. *M. bovis* affects all age groups of cattle (prewean, postwean, neonate and adult) and all cattle sectors such as beef, milk or rearing [3]. *M. bovis* can persist in a herd for very long periods of time, with the possibility of pathogen shedding by the infected animals for a few weeks to several months [13,14]. The evolutionary absence of a cell wall in principle makes *M. bovis* resistant to penicillins and cephalosporins [3,4]. Moreover, in vitro studies on *M. bovis* field isolates show increasing trends in antimicrobial resistance, including tetracyclines and even newer generation macrolides considered effective against *M. bovis* infections [5,15–18]. *M. bovis* infections are usually characterized by chronic course and are difficult to treat successfully [3]. One recent in vivo study has shown an efficacy of treatment of the *M. bovis* pneumonia in calves using enrofloxacin given alone, unlike the combination therapy with co-administration of flunixin meglumine, a nonsteroidal anti-inflammatory drug or pegbovigrastim (immunostimulator), which rather exacerbated the disease. However, it should be remembered that fluoroquinolones, although effective in this case, should be used as antimicrobials of last resort [19]. Some experimental *M. bovis* vaccines have been shown to be immunogenic and protective; however, currently no commercial vaccines are available in Europe with only some autogenous vaccines in use in the United States and Great Britain [20–22].

3. Current Reports on the Epizootic Situation of *M. bovis*

It was previously reported that *M. bovis* has the ability to spread worldwide to countries for a long time considered free of the pathogen because of the widespread international trade in cattle [2,23,24]. The first case of *M. bovis* infection in Finland was recorded relatively recently in 2012 in pneumonic calves. In 2012–2015, 0.26% of Finnish dairy farms were *M. bovis* infected [2]. To date, it is estimated that only 0.8% of Finnish dairy herds were infected with *M. bovis* between 2012 and 2018 [23]. A two-year survey included 19 Finnish dairy farms previously free of *M. bovis* showed mastitis caused by *M. bovis* in over 89% of all farms tested; however, only a few clinical mastitis cases were seen. In the remaining two farms, no *M. bovis* mastitis cases were detected during the study period; calf pneumonia caused by *M. bovis* were, however, observed. In this study, the results may indicate a rather subclinical course of mastitis due to *M. bovis* infection. Additional data including *M. bovis* antibody detection using the MilA ELISA showed the majority of cows were positive for *M. bovis* throughout the study period, regardless of the infection status of the farm. It confirms that *M. bovis* may circulate for long time in the herd [23].

The detection of *M bovis* in New Zealand was remarkable for several reasons. First, New Zealand was probably the last major cattle-rearing nation to become infected; secondly, it does not import cattle, the main route of cross border infection, and had not done so for nearly a decade; and thirdly, New Zealand took the unprecedented decision to eradicate the organism from its cattle industry despite the fact the clinical disease was overwhelmingly mild. *M. bovis* was first detected in a dairy herd at the Bay of Plenty on the South Island in 2017. Since this isolation, up until June 2020, just over 1800 farms have been affected, involving the slaughter of nearly 160,000 cattle at a cost of NZ$203 million (about 116 million euros). With just over 250 farms still affected, complete eradication looks feasible but challenging and would be a first amongst cattle rearing countries. The origins of the outbreaks have still not been definitively traced but whole genome sequencing of 171 isolates from 30 infected herds indicated that the current outbreak was probably caused by recent entry of *M. bovis*, perhaps 1–2 years before detection, from a single source either as a single entry of a single *M. bovis* clone or, potentially, up to three entries of three very closely related *M. bovis* clones from the same source [25]; this suggests that there were probably several simultaneous outbreaks strongly implicating infected imported semen. Indeed *M. bovis* DNA was detected by PCR in one batch of semen but unfortunately could not be isolated. While analyses to date have not identified the source, the most closely related international isolates that have been characterised are European in origin [25].

Interesting information can be gathered by estimating on-farm/within-herd prevalence of *M. bovis* infections [26,27]. Such a repeated cross-sectional six-month study on *M. bovis* intramammary infections was conducted between 2017 and 2018 in four Estonian dairy herds with previously confirmed *M. bovis* positive status. The qPCR results of examination of pooled cow composite milk samples in the four endemically infected herds showed a differential and relatively low within-herd prevalence, which ranged between 0.4% and 12.3%. For the author, this could be a result of the different infection phases, *M. bovis* strain differentiation, intermittent shedding of the pathogen by the infected cows or low concentration of *M. bovis* in the examined milk samples. Similar prevalence (3.7–11%) was observed in clinical cases of mastitis due to *M. bovis* during a six-month study period in the four dairy herds. Additional evaluation of pooled cow colostrum samples during the same study period also showed low prevalence of *M. bovis* in the study herds ranging between 1.7% and 4.7% [26].

Within-herd prevalence of *M. bovis* DNA in cow colostrum samples was also estimated in 2016–2017 in seventeen Belgian herds with a recent infection of *M. bovis*. This survey was performed on dairy, beef and mixed-dairy farms with *M. bovis* positive status diagnosed less than one month before sample collection. The herds were additionally divided into two groups, depending on whether the infection was confirmed only in calves or in both calves and adult animals. The results showed only seven colostrum samples positive for *M. bovis* DNA originated from four herds, which was 1.9% of the total number of samples tested. In the positive farms on-farm/within-herd prevalence ranged between 2.8% and 30.0%, whereas the average within-herd prevalence estimated for all seventeen herds tested was 3.2%. According to the author, the reason for such low average within-herd prevalence of *M. bovis* DNA obtained in this survey was probably a result of differentiation in the infection phases in the periparturient cows or false positive results of real-time PCR assays used in *M. bovis* DNA detection particularly due to the possibility of ongoing co-infections with other *Mycoplasma* species [27]. In 2009, it was reported that 1.5% of all herd tested had bulk tank milk samples positive for *M. bovis* confirmed by culturing and PCR [28].

Data collected in Great Britain between 2006 and 2017 including diagnoses of respiratory disease, mastitis and arthritis due to *M. bovis* infections demonstrated a significant proportion of pneumonia (86.4%), which showed an increasing trend since 2014. The highest number of pneumonia incidents was diagnosed in 2017 (over 120 diagnoses), reaching 7.5% of all diagnosable submissions. For comparison, the annual cases of arthritis and mastitis for all the examined years were less than 30 per year, with a slight predominance for mycoplasma mastitis. In this survey the incidents of *M. bovis* pneumonia were diagnosed mainly in the postwean age group of calves. However, since 2012, the number of pneumonia diagnoses in the preweaning calves was comparable. The smallest number of *M. bovis* pneumonia cases was diagnosed in the neonate age group of calves. Seasonal data collected from 2006 to 2017 showed the largest number of respiratory diagnoses due to *M. bovis* were in the colder seasons, i.e., between October and March, which could be caused not only by temperature fluctuations, but also by closer contact of animals in the herd during housing [20,24]. Temperature fluctuations are probably related to stress accompanied by elevated blood corticosteroid concentrations, which may consequently predispose calves to *M. bovis* infection, as confirmed in both in vivo and in vitro studies using dexamethasone [29–31]. In the remaining months, i.e., from July to September, and from April to June, the respiratory submissions were comparable, although slightly higher in the spring months. Additional examinations also showed a higher incidence of *M. bovis* respiratory disease in the beef sector of cattle (almost 42%). Another slightly less affected cattle sector was dairy with 32.8% of *M. bovis* respiratory submissions [20]. A previous study performed in Great Britain between 1990 and 2000 showed that over 50% of a total of 1413 cattle isolates tested were *M. bovis*, mostly originating from pneumonia cases. *M. bovis* was also isolated from mastitis cases, joint fluid, eyes and sporadically from sheath washings, urogenital tract and heart blood [32].

The problem of subclinical intramammary infections with *M. bovis* as a consequence of recent clinical mastitis outbreaks in four Australian dairy herds was discussed in the study of Hazelton et al., which concluded that an early diagnosis of such cases may consequently prevent the future spread of *M. bovis* in the herd [13]. The apparent cow-level prevalence of *M. bovis* intramammary infections in these herds was determined immediately after cessation of outbreaks. Before the herd sampling between 2014 and 2016 all clinically affected cows due to *M. bovis* were culled. From a total of 2232 cows located in the main milking group of each herd from which 88 initial pooled milk samples were collected, only two *M. bovis* PCR positive cows were detected, which constituted less than 1% of average apparent cow-level prevalence of subclinical intramammary *M. bovis* infection. Additional tests performed individually on 15 cows located in the hospital group of each herd and *M. bovis* suspected gave five positive PCR results. *M. bovis* DNA was also detected by PCR in bulk tank milk collected from two study herds. However, in 6 out of 1813 cows from three study herds, *M. bovis* was isolated using microbiological culture. Five positive culture results were detected in cows located in the hospital group and *M. bovis* suspected, whereas the remaining one was from the main milking group, both within the same herd. For information, the culture positive cow in the main milking group had also positive *M. bovis* PCR result. In addition, *M. bovis* was isolated from bulk tank milk sampled from one study herd; however, it was not the same herd from which *M. bovis* culture positive cows were detected. To estimate *M. bovis* seroprevalence in the four study herds, a total of 199 sera were collected from 50 cows located in the main milking group of each herd, with the exception of one herd from which 49 results were estimated. The results showed the average *M. bovis* seroprevalence of 38%, which varied from 16% to 76%. It is also worth mentioning that in two of the four herds tested, several months after the herd sampling, new clinical cases or positive results in the hospital group bulk tank were reported, both confirmed by *M. bovis* PCR [13].

4. Disease Course and Source of *M. bovis* Infection

M. bovis infections occur with various clinical manifestations, such as pneumonia, mastitis, arthritis, otitis, keratoconjunctivitis, meningitis, endocarditis and others, the most important of which are summarized in Table 1. The clinical picture of respiratory disease diagnosed as *M. bovis* is not usually characteristic and often does not differ from clinical signs caused by infections with other bovine respiratory tract pathogens, especially in the presence of co-infections [20]. The study on feedlot beef calves showed that *M. bovis* was isolated from all diagnosed pneumonia categories, such as caseonecrotic bronchopneumonia, both caseonecrotic and fibrinosuppurative bronchopneumonia or fibrinosuppurative bronchopneumonia alone. In this study distinct synergism in pneumonia cases between *M. bovis* and *Pasteurellaceae* family pathogens, especially for *M. haemolytica,* was demonstrated. Both pathogens were identified in focal coagulative necrosis lesions within lung tissues [33].

In cases of keratoconjunctivitis as well as brain disorders, *M. bovis* infections, which are often overlooked in the differential diagnosis of these diseases, should be taken into account (Table 1).

As recently reported, both clinical and subclinical courses of mastitis due to *M. bovis* infection were detected [13,23]. However, the possibility of subclinical intramammary infections with *M. bovis* as a consequence of the recent clinical mastitis outbreaks should be considered as previously presented in the Section 3 in the study of Hazelton et al. [13].

It was first recognized that *M. bovis*-positive semen used in artificial insemination was a cause of mastitis outbreak in two naive dairy herds, despite high biosecurity and good farming practice carried out on these farms [2]. Out of the total of ten bulls used to inseminate cows with *M. bovis* mastitis diagnosed, only one of them appeared to be the *M. bovis* carrier. Additionally, only one of the cows from each herd that were inseminated with the contaminated processed semen from the same bull developed mastitis. In both study herds, the infection not only transmitted to other cows that were not inseminated with *M. bovis*-positive semen, but also to calves. The core-genome multilocus sequence typing (cgMLST) analysis of *M. bovis* strains isolated from the mastitis cases and the bull semen clustered together [2].

Table 1. Examples of clinical manifestations of *M. bovis* infections. The sequence presented is consistent with the frequency of each clinical manifestation from the most to the least frequently diagnosed cases in cattle.

Course of *M. bovis* Infection	Type of Research (Experimental/Survey)	Cattle Sector	Main Clinical Signs/Lesions/Subclinical	Methods Used for the Infection Confirmation/Presence	Reference
pneumonia	survey	beef	caseonecrotic bronchopneumonia; fibrinosuppurative bronchopneumonia	IHC; PCR	[33]
	experimental	dairy-cross	nasal discharge; coughing; caseonecrotic pneumonia	ELISA for *M. bovis* antigen detection; IHC; ELISA for specific antibody detection	[19]
mastitis	survey	dairy	clinical mastitis; subclinical mastitis	culture; real-time PCR; two different ELISAs for specific antibody detection (MilA IgG ELISA; BioX ELISA)	[23]
	survey		clinical mastitis; subclinical mastitis	culture; PCR; ELISA for specific antibody detection	[13]
arthritis	survey	beef	arthritis; tenosynovitis	culture; passive hemagglutination test	[33]
	experimental	dairy	joint swelling; lameness/fibrinosuppurative synovitis and tenosynovitis; thrombus presence	culture; indirect hemagglutination test	[34]
otitis	survey	dairy	ear droop; otic exudate	ELISA for specific antibody detection; DGGE	[35]
	survey	beef	ear droop; exudative otitis media; facial paralysis; occasionally nasal exudate; nystagmus, head tilt, ataxia/suppurative lesions in the middle ear; lung consolidation (most cases); cerebellar meningitis (some cases)	culturing; immune-peroxidase test; PCR; IHC; transmission electron microscopy	[7]
kerato-conjunctivitis	survey	beef	"pink eye" signs	culture; RAPD; PCR-RFLP; DNA sequencing	[8]
brain disorders	survey	dairy	head tilt; central nervous system signs/purulent meningitis	ELISA for specific antibody detection	[36]
			lethargy, blindness; teeth grinding/cerebral hemisphere necrosis	enrichment and capture ELISA	
endocarditis	survey	beef	no clinical signs; caseated lesions in the heart	culture; *uvrC* gene PCR; loop-mediated isothermal amplification assay; IHC	[10]

The role of airborne transmission of *M. bovis* is unclear with little experimental evidence supporting this route of infection [37,38]. In response to exposure of calves to aerosolized *M. bovis*, respiratory disease was induced. In the infected calves, specific *M. bovis* lung lesions confirmed by necropsy and histological examinations were observed despite the lack of clinical signs. However, re-isolation of *M. bovis* from the upper trachea in most infected calves was additional confirmation of this infection route [37].

Recent reports on *M. bovis* indicated colostrum as a possible source of infection based on positive results for *M. bovis* DNA [26,27]. Additionally, in one of these studies, herd-specific *M. bovis* strains were isolated from cows with clinical mastitis and calves affected with respiratory disease showing possible transmission of the pathogen between dairy cows and calves via contaminated milk. However, in this study other routes of *M. bovis* infection transmission like direct/indirect contact between animals within the study herds, animal handling or air-borne route cannot be excluded [26]. The most important sources of *M. bovis* infection/routes of *M. bovis* infection transmission are summarized in Table 2. Other no less important sources/routes of *M. bovis* infection transmission not included in the Table 2 such as nose-to-nose contact between animals or fomites (e.g., farm-personnel's contaminated hands, equipment), although difficult to directly prove or document, should also be considered [26,39,40].

Within the host, *M. bovis* disseminates by the haematogenous route, which may result in subsequent lesions in organs other than those initially affected. In one such study all diagnosed cases of arthritis in feedlot beef calves were accompanied by lung lesions, which accounted for nearly 50% of all diagnosed *M. bovis*-related pneumonias. The arthritis cases were probably of pulmonary origin [33]. In post-mortem findings in *M. bovis* affected calves, both meningitis and otitis media/interna were diagnosed. In other calf necropsy examinations, necrosis within the brain and fibrinous heart lesions due to *M. bovis* infection were evident [36]. The ability of *M. bovis* to spread within different organs of the same host was previously confirmed [7]. In the majority of calves diagnosed with suppurative otitis media severe lung lesions were observed. In some of them cerebellar meningitis was also diagnosed. Additionally, in some calves, *M. bovis* antigen was identified in the temporal bone, liver and kidney [7].

Table 2. Examples of sources of *M. bovis* infection/routes of *M. bovis* infection transmission.

Source of Infection/Route of Infection Transmission	Type of Research (Experimental/Survey)	Cattle Sector	Number of Herd/Farms Tested	Methods Used for the Infection Confirmation/Detection	Reference
colostrum	survey	dairy	4	qPCR	[26]
	survey	dairy, beef and dairy-mixed	17	real-time PCR	[27]
milk	survey	dairy	4	qPCR; culturing; core-genome multilocus sequence typing (cgMLST)	[26]
semen	survey	dairy	2	culturing; real-time PCR; WGS; cgMLST analysis	[2]
air-borne	experimental	dairy-cross	not applicable	culturing; *polC* PCR; MilA IgG ELISA; *post mortem* examination; histopathological examination	[37]
intrauterine	survey	dairy	not described	culturing; IHC; ISH	[41]

5. Currently Used Diagnostic Methods

The clinical signs of infections in cattle associated with *M. bovis* are non-specific; for that reason, sensitive, accurate and rapid testing of animals is needed for reliable diagnosis. Culturing of *M. bovis* is a gold standard method but is time-consuming and requires specific conditions. Different kinds of media are widely used in experimental studies and in confirmation of infection caused by *M. bovis*, and include Hayflick's [42], modified PPLO [43] and Eaton's [44]. Mycoplasmas are fastidious, slow growing and can be easily overgrown by other bacteria. During the last few years various tests have been used for the detection of *M. bovis* infections in cattle (Table 3).

Table 3. The characteristics of recently developed methods for *M. bovis* detection in various specimens from cattle.

Assay/Target	Samples	Limit of Detection	Sensitivity	Specificity	Reference
real-time PCR/*uvr*C	lung samples (n = 30); milk samples (n = 21)	100 fg DNA; 40 genome copies/reaction; 250 CFU/mL	10^3-fold more sensitive than conventional PCR	100% (evaluated for 6 *Mycoplasma* spp. and 6 species of bacteria)	[45]
qPCR/*uvr*C	deep nasopharyngeal swabs (n = 208)	1.61×10^2 CFU/mL	100%	87.27%	[46]
qPCR/*gltX*	milk samples from individual quarters (n = 9); bulk tank milk samples (n = 59)	10–100 genome equivalents/reaction; 1×10^4–1×10^5 cells/mL	100%	94.4% (evaluated for 3 *Mycoplasma* spp.)	[47]

real-time multiplex PCR
*M. bovis/uvr*C
*M. californicum/rpo*B
M. bovigenitalium/16S–23S rRNA
	swab samples (n = 95);
	semen samples (n = 44);
	individual milk samples (n = 114);
	bulk tank milk samples (n = 221)
		1.3×10^2–1.3×10^7 CFU/mL	not applicable	100%
				(evaluated for 10 *Mycoplasma* spp. and 11 species of bacteria)
					[48]

multiplex qPCR Pneumo 4B/*M. bovis* *M. haemolytica* *P. multocida* *H. somni*	tracheal aspirate samples (n = 176)	10 genome copies; 1.1–3.3 $\log_{10}$ CFU/0.5 mL	0.96	0.71 (evaluated for 6 *Mycoplasma* spp. and 66 species of bacteria)	[49]
multiplex qPCR Mastit 4/*M. bovis* *Staphylococcus aureus* *Streptococcus agalactiae* *Streptococcus uberis*	milk samples	-	-	-	[26]
real-time multiplex RPA/*M. bovis/uvr*C *M. haemolytica/nmaA*	deep nasopharyngeal swabs (n = 100)	40 genome copies/reaction	-	98.0 (evaluated for 10 *Mycoplasma* spp. and 35 species of bacteria)	[50]
real-time multiplex PCR PathoProof™ Mastitis Major 4.2/*M. bovis* *Staphylococcus aureus* *Streptococcus agalactiae* *Streptococcus uberis*	milk samples	-	-	-	[13]

Table 3. *Cont.*

Assay/Target	Samples	Limit of Detection	Sensitivity	Specificity	Reference
real-time PCR VetMAX™ *M. bovis*	tissue samples, bronchoalveolar lavage fluid samples, synovial fluid, milk samples	10 genome copies/reaction	100%	100% (evaluated for 50 other bacteria species, including *M. agalactiae*, *Streptococcus uberis* and *Streptococcus dysgalactiae*	[27]
LAMP/*uvr*C, *gyr*B	milk samples from 95 dairy farms	5×10^1 CFU/mL	96.8%–100%	94.7%–100% (evaluated for 2 *Mycoplasma* spp. and 4 species of bacteria)	[51]
LAMP/*opp*D	milk samples from individual quarters (n = 9); bulk tank milk samples (n = 59)	10 genome equivalents/reaction; 1×10^4 cells/mL	87.5%	82.4% (evaluated for 3 *Mycoplasma* spp.)	[47]
PURE-LAMP not applicable	bulk tank milk samples (n = 12); mature milk samples (n = 73); colostrum/transitional milk samples (n = 74); mastitis milk samples (n = 122)	$>10^2$ CFU/mL of milk	57.0%–97.0%	100% (evaluated for 5 *Mycoplasma* spp.)	[52]
RPA-LFD/*uvr*C, *opp*D-*opp*F	nasal swab samples (n = 288); fresh lung samples (n = 80); joint fluid samples (n = 32); bulk tank milk samples (n = 42)	20 genome copies/reaction	99.0%	95.61% (evaluated for 10 *Mycoplasma* spp. and 13 species of bacteria)	[53]
MALDI-TOF MS	culture-enriched bronchoalveolar lavage fluid samples (n = 104)	not applicable	86.6%	86.4%	[54]

5.1. Real-Time PCR Assays for *M. bovis* Detection

Detection of *M. bovis* by real-time PCR preceded by culture enrichment of the samples improves detection when DNA is present at low concentrations. Furthermore, a selective broth-enrichment step increases the probability of *Mycoplasma* recovery when compared to direct plating on agar [55]. In the real-time PCR assay [45], milk samples from dairies and lung tissue samples were culture-enriched in PPLO broth for 24 h before analysis. In another qPCR for *M. bovis* testing [46], the nasopharyngeal swabs were cultured for 3–5 days before the analysis. The molecular methods are optimized for the detection of *M. bovis* in nasopharyngeal swabs and milk samples, but they can be optimized to be used for the detection of *M. bovis* in different specimens [2,26,27,48,49]. In 2020, a qPCR was developed for the detection of *M. bovis* in tracheal aspirate samples derived from calves [49]. In research on *M. bovis* intramammary infection, the presence of this pathogen in colostrum and additionally in milk from clinical cases was assessed with qPCR [26]. It is also possible to detect *M. bovis* in processed semen [2,48]. The real-time PCR assays are characterised often by a low limit of detection (LOD) and specificity near to 100% [45–48]. Taking into consideration that the number of mycoplasmas that are shed during the infection is about $>1 \times 10^6$ CFU/mL in milk [4] and the LOD for real-time PCR for *M. bovis* detection in milk is 1.3×10^2 CFU/mL [48], the probability of the detection of infected cow in a herd is high. To assess the best sensitivity, the real-time PCR assays for *M. bovis* detection are usually used after an enrichment procedure of the samples. Additionally, centrifugation of the milk and plating the resuspended pellet of bacteria improves detection of mycoplasmas with culture. After such treatment, it was four times more likely to detect of a positive sample when compared to traditional culture regarding very small concentrations [56]. The combination of culture of viable bacteria and qPCR results enables the most accurate confirmation of active infection in animals.

5.2. Fast and Cost-Effective Assays for *M. bovis* Detection

Another approach for *M. bovis* detection is to design a simple and cost-effective assay run at a single temperature without the need of using specific equipment, which will be useful to process in developing countries. LAMP is recently of interest because it enables results to be received quickly, and the reaction is normally completed in less than 2 h; furthermore, there is no need to have expensive laboratory equipment, as it is performed at a single temperature [57]. LAMP gives better results than qPCR when performed on purified DNA but is susceptible to contamination. Two assays, namely LAMP and qPCR developed for *M. bovis* detection in milk samples from individual cow quarters and bulk tank milk samples, accurately detected *M. bovis* isolates but gave false positive results for one *Mycoplasma bovigenitalium* isolate [47]. Another method called isothermal DNA amplification assay, a technique based on recombinase polymerase amplification (RPA) with lateral flow dipstick (LFD), allows one to obtain the result in 30 min and is dedicated for *M. bovis* DNA extracted directly from clinical samples i.e., nasal swabs, lungs tissue samples, joint fluids and bulk tank milk samples; no cross-reactions were observed with other *Mycoplasma* species [53]. Usually, LAMP assays are more sensitive than end-point PCRs, for example high sensitivity and specificity for all milk sample types was obtained with the use of LAMP combined with a procedure for ultra-rapid extraction (PURE-LAMP), in which various sample types i.e., bulk tank milk, mature milk, colostrum/transitional milk and mastitis milk were examined [52]. Similar parameters were obtained in LAMP for the examination of *M. bovis* in milk from mastitis cases [51].

5.3. Immunohistochemistry and In-Situ Hybridization

Although molecular methods are advantageous, they can only provide the data on *M. bovis* DNA, and there is lacking information about the presence of viable bacteria. Immunohistochemistry (IHC) and in-situ hybridization (ISH) are types of techniques which have the advantage that they are able to detect the localization of *M. bovis* antigen or DNA, respectively, in the examined tissue of the infected animals [12,19,41,58,59]. The IHC used in the study on calves experimentally infected with

M. bovis allows one to detect *M. bovis* antigen in the bronchiolar epithelial cells in the lung tissue with histopathological changes that are characteristic for bronchiolitis [19]. Results of another experiment proved that *M. bovis* antigen was detected on the surface and inside the cytoplasm of bronchiolar epithelial cells in the pneumonic foci and in the cytoplasm of phagocytes at the margin of bronchiolar exudates [58]. In the study on aborted foetus and neonatal calf that were infected with *M. bovis*, its antigen was found with the use of IHC in the brain, liver, lungs and placenta of aborted foetus, and ISH showed the presence of its DNA i.e., in lungs and placenta of the examined animals [41]. The research on long-term survival of *M. bovis* in tissues of infected calves showed the persistence of this pathogen in necrotic lung lesions several weeks after the infection with the use of both methods [59]. It is also possible to examine the pulmonary samples of calves with BRD. IHC was used to detect the *M. bovis* antigen intralesional in different areas of the lungs [12]. However, while these techniques allow one to obtain significant information, they are also expensive and labour intensive and require trained staff.

5.4. A Matrix-Assisted Laser Desorption/Ionization Time-of-Flight Mass Spectrometry for M. bovis Detection

The matrix-assisted laser desorption/ionization time-of-flight mass spectrometry (MALDI-TOF MS) procedure has been applied to *M. bovis* detection. It was optimised for the detection of *M. bovis* isolates and found to be a suitable test for routine diagnostics in cattle, especially those from BRD cases. The protocol enables the identification of *M. bovis* from bronchoalveolar lavage fluid (BALF) after enrichment in culture. The higher number of positive samples was obtained after 72 h of enrichment. The main advantage of MALDI-TOF MS is that it only detects viable bacteria, which indicates that cattle have active rather than historic infections [54].

5.5. Molecular Typing

The analysis of *M. bovis* isolates with typing and sequencing methods can give additional information about their relationships and evolution. The multilocus sequence typing (MLST) analysis was proved to be suitable for molecular typing of *M. bovis* and the assessment of geographical relatedness of isolates. The MLST scheme based on eleven housekeeping genes was evaluated. Three genes, *dnaN*, *metS* and *hsp70*, were taken for the sequence analysis and the remaining eight genes, i.e., *adk*, *efp*, *gmk*, *gyrB*, *polC*, *rpoB*, *tpiA* and *uvrC* were not chosen for the further analysis. It allows the acquiring of information on sequence variation, its type of distribution and disappearance of some sequence types [60]. A later study [61] assessed two MLST schemes for *M. bovis* isolate typing. The comparison of the performance of the two MLST schemes and additional identification of a new reference scheme capable of full typing of the examined isolates was made. The PubMLST reference method contains *adh-1*, *gltX*, *gspA*, *gyrA*, *gyrB*, *pta-2*, *tdk* and *tkt* locus; it is thought to be discriminatory and informative enough, but in this study, *adh-1*, one of the typing loci of *M. bovis* isolates, was missed. According to this reference scheme, the *adh-1* locus should be retired from the analysis. This approach was not beneficial for the study because the discrimination index received with the use of the six remaining PubMLST loci failed to reach the benchmark recommended for a reference method, and the addition of a seventh locus had to be made. The alternative scheme contains seven loci: *aptA*, *dnaA*, *metS*, *recA*, *rpoD*, *tkt* and *tufA*. The comparisons of examined *M. bovis* genome sequences identified the *dnaA* locus from the alternative scheme as the optimal replacement for *adh-1*.

Another approach for epidemiological studies is the use of whole genome sequencing (WGS) to evaluate the molecular epidemiology and genomic diversity of *M. bovis* isolates as well as their genetic relationship. The single nucleotide polymorphism (SNP) analysis can be used to assess the intraspecies relationship and the presence of a dominant genotype that can be associated with one type of disease. This study is relevant to better understand the global epidemiology of this important pathogen and to assess control strategies [62]. Comparison of the *M. bovis* sequences can be used in assessing the genetic diversity of the strains [63] or to get the information about gene virulence [64].

WGS was used in New Zealand to track the outbreaks first identified in 2017. In all, 171 isolates from 30 infected herds have so far been sequenced, and results indicate that the current outbreak was probably caused by recent entry of the mycoplasma, perhaps 1–2 years before detection, from a single source either as a single border crossing of a single clone or, potentially, up to three border crossings of three very closely related clones from the same source (TAG 2019) probably in germplasm imported from Europe.

5.6. Serological Approaches

Serological diagnosis based on detection of specific antibodies to *M. bovis* is suitable and practical for the assessment of prevalence and epidemiological studies of herds [39]. Although serological testing is a reliable method for identification of infected animals, specific antibodies do not appear until 10 to 14 days after the infection but remain elevated for several months [65]. Various indirect ELISAs are used for anti-*M. bovis* antibody detection in cattle herds. The BIO K302 ELISA (BioX Diagnostics) was applied for evaluation of antibody response to *M. bovis* in serum and milk samples [13,66,67]. A study conducted in Belgium [67] showed that the ELISA is able to detect *M. bovis* specific antibodies in bulk tank milk up to 12 months after the outbreak of the disease. Researchers [66] examined bulk milk tank samples for all Danish herds with this ELISA and concluded that the cut-off value should be increased from 37%, as suggested for animal-level diagnosis, to 50%, to obtain more adequate sensitivity and specificity for bulk tank milk analysis. On the other hand, as a result of a European inter-laboratory comparison conducted on 180 serum samples, the sensitivity and specificity of BIO K302 ELISA was determined to be 49.1% and 89.6%, respectively [68]. However, in 2020 it was confirmed that this ELISA was suitable for the serological evaluation of anti-*M. bovis* antibodies in longitudinal studies. Despite the low number of apparent clinical mastitis cases, it was useful in evaluation of *M. bovis* seroprevalence in dairy herds, which was on average 38% (16–76%), as mentioned before [13].

Another indirect ELISA, made in-house and based on a fragment of a recombinant mycoplasma immunogenic lipase A (MilA), was developed [69]. This assay can be also useful for bulk tank milk sample analysis. The results of the presence of anti-*M. bovis* antibodies in bulk tank milk were positively correlated with the antibody detection in sera of the examined animals. Additionally, there was made a comparison between BIO K 260 (BioX Diagnostics) and the MilA ELISA [23], and the latter test gave a higher number of positive samples for *M. bovis*, and they were more convergent with those obtained with culture or real-time PCR. The obtained sensitivity and specificity for this test was 94.3% and 94.4%, respectively. Additionally, it was shown that the MilA ELISA is also suitable for testing the presence of anti-*M. bovis* antibodies in the early stages of calf life (from the 3rd week of life) [70].

5.7. Interlaboratory Trials of Diagnostic Tests

M. bovis causes serious health problems in cattle herds almost all over the world, but its detection is not harmonised as yet and relies on different diagnostic methods, often in-house molecular techniques based on a variety of target genes and various different DNA extraction methods. There was conducted a European interlaboratory comparison of the diagnostic utility of the molecular tests for *M. bovis* detection [71]. Six laboratories from different countries were included in the study. Five different DNA extraction methods from bacterial culture and BALF samples were used. The molecular tests were made with the use of seven different PCR assays based on *polC*, *oppD*, *uvrC* and V4-V4 16S rRNA target genes. The comparison revealed that although the research used various assays, they had comparable diagnostic utility for *M. bovis* detection in cattle. The analytical specificity of the different PCR methods was comparable for all of the laboratories, except one, where *M. agalactiae* was detected because of the use of 16S rRNA target gene. The LOD was from 10 to 10^3 for the real-time, and from 10^3 to 10^6 CFU/mL for the end-point assays. According to the authors, this difference was acceptable. Cultures correctly detected the presence of *M. bovis* in bronchoalveolar lavage fluid samples and were consistent with PCR results. The recent comparison of diagnostic methods used in the different veterinary laboratories fortunately showed consensus.

5.8. Mixed Infections

Other *Mycoplasma* spp. can also be associated with *M. bovis* infections in cattle. In BRD cases, most often *M. dispar*, *M. canis* and *M. arginini* are implicated [3,72]. In mastitis mycoplasmatica and reproductive disorders, *M. bovigenitalium*, *M. californicum* and *M. alkalescens* can also participate [73,74]. A test based on PCR with the 16SrRNA target gene and separation of the PCR products using denaturing gradient gel electrophoresis (PCR–DGGE) enabled the differentiation of 13 *Mycoplasma* spp. of bovine origin in mixed infections [75]. Traditionally, culture is used for the confirmation of BRD infections, but the incubation period for each examined bacterial pathogens is different and samples inoculated onto agar plates are often overgrown with other, fast growing bacteria. For that reason, the multiplex real-time PCRs used by the laboratories [49,50,76] are the most suitable for simultaneous direct detection of *M. bovis* and other pathogens involved in BRD, such as *P. multocida*, *M. haemolytica* and *H. somni*, in contrast to methods not dedicated for different pathogen identification in mixed infections such as one-target PCR, traditional culture or MALDI-TOF MS [77]. When using one target PCR, there is no information about the involvement of other pathogens in the disease, different bacteria have various growth requirements and slow growing bacteria can be easily overgrown by others, and MALDI-TOF MS is not able properly detect all organisms from polymicrobial samples.

Various diagnostics methods for fast and accurate detection of *M. bovis* in various sample types and typing methods for identification and analysis of its strains in the last few years have been developed for evaluation of the disease course. Methods should be chosen according to the purpose of the survey, for herd-level testing or for individuals, or should be considered in terms of its usage for the specimen. The use of a combination of molecular, serological and culture-based methods is necessary for reliable diagnosis of diseases caused by this pathogen in cattle.

6. Control—Recommendations for *M. bovis* Control Programs

Due to the lack of efficient vaccines against *M. bovis* and increasing trends in antimicrobial resistance of *M. bovis* field isolates, it is important to provide consistent, possibly unified rules for effective control and/or eradication of *M. bovis* infections. However, in many ways, preventing the spread of *M bovis* into healthy herds is relatively easy, as the screening of small numbers of cattle from source herds by serological tests, such as ELISA, can ensure that herds remain free of disease; this was successfully achieved in the Republic of Ireland when the national herd free of *M. bovis* was restocked following the BSE crisis [78]. Whether the Irish national herd is still free is unknown. However, few countries have active eradication plans for *M. bovis*, and because of its presence in all cattle-rearing countries, it is not subject to OIE regulations; indeed, it is very difficult for countries to impose trade restrictions when they themselves are infected. Israel has attempted to identify countries that export infected livestock into their country by mass screening between 2010–2011 and found cattle from Lithuania, Hungary and Australia to be highly seropositive [79].

Undoubtedly the most ambitious and unique plan for the complete eradication of *M. bovis* was made in New Zealand where infection was first recognised in 2017. The decision was made to cull infected and contact cattle when the number of infected farms was low but now remains increasingly challenging though still feasible according to Technical Advisory Group in 2019 [25] because of the high number of infected farms traced subsequently. To date over 2000 infected farms have been traced, although most without clinical or gross pathological signs. Detecting infected farms proved difficult at first because of the use of relatively insensitive diagnostic tests, but now serological ELISA testing bulk tank milk is being used in parallel with real-time PCRs. This has increased confidence that eradication can be achieved, although the process is likely to take at least 5 years or maybe longer.

In Finland, there is a voluntary *M. bovis* control program (Animal Health ETT) for cattle farms since 2013, which four years later associated 75% of all dairy farms [2,23].

Pasteurisation or heat treatment is one of proposals to eliminate the risk of *M. bovis* shedding via colostrum or raw milk. Another alternative may be to avoid pooling of colostrum within endemically infected farms, discarding colostrum originating from *M. bovis* affected cows, or colostrum purchasing as replacer [27]. As previously documented, a commercial on-farm pasteurizer was able to destroy *Mycoplasma* spp. tested in 71.7 °C for 15 s, including *M. bovis*. Additional data showed an average 25% reduction in total immunoglobulin concentration in colostrum after 30 min pasteurization, from 22% at the low temperature range (63.9–66.7 °C) to 27% at high temperatures (68.3–70.8 °C) [80]. However, heat treatment of colostrum may affect cytokine absorption and immune response in neonatal calves. A reduction in the circulating IL-1β in dairy calves fed colostrum heat-treated to 60 °C for 60 min was demonstrated, although without affecting other immune parameters tested such as IFN-γ or IgG concentrations [81].

The generally recommended rule to control subclinical intramammary infections due to *M. bovis* is sampling of cows with high somatic cell counts (SCC) in milk; however, as was shown in some studies, cows with no clinical signs of mastitis and low SCCs (<200,000 cells/mL) can be *M. bovis* positive [13,82]. However, these differences may be a result of the disease stage. The study of Kauf et al. [83] showed that infusion of a mastitic *M. bovis* strain in one quarter of ten first-lactation cows with milk SCCs of <200,000 cells/mL caused initial increase in mean milk SCCs within 66 h post infusion. During the study period, the SCC counts fluctuated, with a peak value of 119.82×10^6 cells/mL at 90 h following the infusion; however, they persisted at a higher level than the control until the end of the study at 240 h post infection [83].

It was recommended that clinically affected *M. bovis* cows should be separated and moved from the main milking group to hospital or another group to prevent the infection spread in the herd. According to the author's opinion, cows within main milking group should be constantly monitored via bulk tank milk testing [13]. However, there was evidence of *M. bovis* mastitis incidence and transmission in the hospital pen following the introduction of cows with *M. bovis* clinical mastitis from three different milking pens, which should not be underestimated [84]. Bulk tank milk testing seems to be effective due to previously reported mycoplasma shedding via milk of cows with mastitis at above 1×10^6 CFU/mL [4]. It was suggested that if a positive result is obtained in bulk tank milk testing, it is a good strategy to follow up with pooled milk samples from five cows to identify the individuals [85]. However, SCC screening in bulk tank milk for *M. bovis* infection control does not appear to be effective [13]. An important suggestion for programs designed for *M. bovis* mastitis control is milk testing of newly introduced animals into the lactating herd. Additionally, using antibiotics to treat *M. bovis* mastitis should be discouraged [4].

One recommendation for *M. bovis* control programs is to combine regular monitoring of mastitic cows and pneumonia calves with bulk tank milk testing and longitudinal screening of young stock in herds [23].

Another option in the prevention/eradication of *M. bovis* infections is farm sanitization using effective disinfectants. Only a few studies on disinfectant efficacy in inactivating *M. bovis* has been undertaken. The most recent study estimated the efficacy of different dilutions of citric acid and sodium hypochlorite against *M. bovis*. The results showed that the acceptance criterion for an effective disinfectant of 10^6 fold reduction in the *M. bovis* viability was met for 0.5% citric acid and 1% sodium hypochlorite in the presence of organic material. However, in the absence of organic material, a 10^6 fold reduction in the *M. bovis* viability was observed for 0.25% citric acid and 0.04% sodium hypochlorite [86]. In another study, the efficacy of five different classes of teat dips were tested against *M. bovis* in the context of their use in maintaining pre- and post-milking hygiene and preventing *M. bovis* mastitis. All of them showed germicidal activity against *M. bovis*, but the iodine-based formulation was the most effective in this study [87].

To reduce the risk of *M. bovis* shedding in semen, it is worth paying more attention to the type and volume of antibiotics added to seminal extenders, because currently used mixtures have a more bacteriostatic rather than bactericidal effect on *M. bovis*. According to the author, the antibiotic combination in seminal extenders should be re-evaluated or alternatively *M. bovis* testing in processed semen should be performed [2].

Above all, it is important to recognize the subclinically infected cattle, which can be facilitated by regular monitoring/screening of different age groups of animals using various methods to prevent uncontrolled *M. bovis* shedding [23].

In summary, *M. bovis* infections are difficult to control/eradicate most of all due to the intracellular nature of the pathogen and biofilm production, which effectively hamper disease treatment. Additionally, increasing trends in antimicrobial resistance of field *M. bovis* isolates reduce the effectiveness of the therapy used routinely for *M. bovis* infections. The high genetic and antigenic variability of field *M. bovis* strains makes them easier to avoid the host immune response. In addition, the general chronic nature of the disease facilitates the spread of the mycoplasma in the herd. Additionally, the lack of effective vaccines makes the eradication of *M. bovis* infections very difficult from cattle population. The relentless and silent spread of *M. bovis* into the infection-free areas is also a feature of this disease. Therefore, regular monitoring/screening of different age groups of animals should be applied, especially for early detection of subclinical carriers in cattle herds; work is also required to develop effective vaccines to provide suitable control of *M. bovis* infections. Finally, there is also an urgent need to develop uniform recommendations that will be included in the programs designed for *M. bovis* infection control.

Author Contributions: Conceptualization, K.D.; writing—original draft preparation, K.D., R.A.J.N., E.S.; writing—review and editing, D.B. All authors have read and agreed to the published version of the manuscript.

Funding: This research received no external funding.

Conflicts of Interest: The authors declare no conflict of interest.

References

1. Ministry for Primary Industries. First Case of Mycoplasma Bovis Found in Bay of Plenty. 2017. Available online: https://www.tvnz.co.nz/one-news/new-zealand/first-case-mycoplasma-bovis-found-in-bay-plenty (accessed on 20 June 2020).
2. Haapala, V.; Pohjanvirta, T.; Vähänikkilä, N.; Halkilahti, J.; Simonen, H.; Pelkonen, S.; Soveri, T.; Simojoki, H.; Autio, T. Semen as a source of *Mycoplasma bovis* mastitis in dairy herds. *Vet. Microbiol.* **2018**, *216*, 60–66. [CrossRef] [PubMed]
3. Nicholas, R.; Ayling, R.; McAuliffe, L. *Mycoplasma Diseases of Ruminants*, 1st ed.; CABI Publishing: Oxford, UK, 2008.
4. Nicholas, R.A.J.; Fox, L.K.; Lysnyansky, I. Mycoplasma mastitis in cattle: To cull or not to cull. *Vet. J.* **2016**, *216*, 142–147. [CrossRef] [PubMed]
5. Klein, U.; de Jong, A.; Youala, M.; El Garch, F.; Stevenin, C.; Moyaert, H.; Rose, M.; Catania, S.; Gyuranecz, M.; Pridmore, A.; et al. New antimicrobial susceptibility data from monitoring of *Mycoplasma bovis* isolated in Europe. *Vet. Microbiol.* **2019**, *238*, 108432. [CrossRef] [PubMed]
6. Houlihan, M.G.; Veenstra, B.; Christian, M.K.; Nicholas, R.; Ayling, R. Mastitis and arthritis in two dairy herds caused by *Mycoplasma bovis*. *Vet. Rec.* **2007**, *160*, 126–127. [CrossRef]
7. Maeda, T.; Shibahara, T.; Kimura, K.; Wada, Y.; Sato, K.; Imada, Y.; Ishikawa, Y.; Kadota, K. *Mycoplasma bovis*-associated suppurative otitis media and pneumonia in bull calves. *J. Comp. Pathol.* **2003**, *129*, 100–110. [CrossRef]
8. Alberti, A.; Filippa Addis, M.; Chessa, B.; Cubeddu, T.; Profiti, M.; Rosati, S.; Ruiu, A.; Pittau, M. Molecular and antigenic characterization of a *Mycoplasma bovis* strain causing an outbreak of infectious keratoconjunctivitis. *J. Vet. Diagn. Invest.* **2006**, *18*, 41–51. [CrossRef]
9. Kinde, H.; Daft, B.M.; Walker, R.L.; Charlton, B.R.; Petty, R. *Mycoplasma bovis* associated with decubital abscesses in Holstein calves. *J. Vet. Diagn. Invest.* **1993**, *5*, 194–197. [CrossRef]
10. Kanda, T.; Tanaka, S.; Suwanruengsri, M.; Sukmawinata, E.; Uemura, R.; Yamaguchi, R.; Sueyoshi, M. Bovine Endocarditis Associated with *Mycoplasma bovis*. *J. Comp. Pathol.* **2019**, *171*, 53–58. [CrossRef]
11. Pardon, B.; Callens, J.; Maris, J.; Allais, L.; Van Praet, W.; Deprez, P.; Ribbens, S. Pathogen-specific risk factors in acute outbreaks of respiratory disease in calves. *J. Dairy Sci.* **2020**, *103*, 2556–2566. [CrossRef]

12. Oliveira, T.E.S.; Pelaquim, I.F.; Flores, E.F.; Massi, R.P.; Valdiviezo, M.J.J.; Pretto-Giordano, L.G.; Alfieri, A.A.; Saut, J.P.E.; Headley, S.A. *Mycoplasma bovis* and viral agents associated with the development of bovine respiratory disease in adult dairy cows. *Transbound. Emerg. Dis.* **2019**, *67*, 82–93. [CrossRef]
13. Hazelton, M.S.; Morton, J.M.; Parker, A.M.; Sheehy, P.A.; Bosward, K.L.; Malmo, J.; House, J.K. Whole dairy herd sampling to detect subclinical intramammary *Mycoplasma bovis* infection after clinical mastitis outbreaks. *Vet. Microbiol.* **2020**, *244*, 108662. [CrossRef] [PubMed]
14. Punyapornwithaya, V.; Fox, L.K.; Hancock, D.D.; Gay, J.M.; Alldredge, J.R. Association between an outbreak strain causing mycoplasma bovis mastitis and its asymptomatic carriage in the herd: A case study from Idaho, USA. *Prev. Vet. Med.* **2010**, *93*, 66–70. [CrossRef] [PubMed]
15. Ayling, R.D.; Rosales, R.S.; Barden, G.; Gosney, F.L. Changes in antimicrobial susceptibility of *Mycoplasma bovis* isolates from Great Britain. *Vet. Rec.* **2014**, *175*, 486. [CrossRef] [PubMed]
16. Gautier-Bouchardon, A.V.; Ferré, S.; Le Grand, D.; Paoli, A.; Gay, E.; Poumarat, F. Overall decrease in the susceptibility of *Mycoplasma bovis* to antimicrobials over the past 30 years in France. *PLoS ONE* **2014**, *9*, e87672. [CrossRef]
17. Sulyok, K.M.; Kreizinger, Z.; Fekete, L.; Hrivnák, V.; Magyar, T.; Jánosi, S.; Schweitzer, N.; Turcsányi, I.; Makrai, L.; Erdélyi, K.; et al. Antibiotic susceptibility profiles of *Mycoplasma bovis* strains isolated from cattle in Hungary, Central Europe. *BMC Vet. Res.* **2014**, *10*, 256. [CrossRef]
18. Ayling, R.D.; Baker, S.E.; Peek, M.L.; Simon, A.J.; Nicholas, R.A.J. Comparison of in vitro activity of danofloxacin, florfenicol, oxytetracycline, spectinomycin and tilmicosin against recent field isolates of *Mycoplasma bovis*. *Vet. Rec.* **2000**, *146*, 745–747. [CrossRef]
19. Dudek, K.; Bednarek, D.; Ayling, R.D.; Kycko, A.; Reichert, M. Preliminary study on the effects of enrofloxacin, flunixin meglumine and pegbovigrastim on *Mycoplasma bovis* pneumonia. *BMC Vet. Res.* **2019**, *15*, 371. [CrossRef]
20. Ridley, A.; Hateley, G. *Mycoplasma bovis* investigations in cattle. *Vet. Rec.* **2018**, *183*, 256–258.
21. Dudek, K.; Bednarek, D.; Ayling, R.D.; Kycko, A.; Szacawa, E.; Karpińska, T.A. An experimental vaccine composed of two adjuvants gives protection against *Mycoplasma bovis* in calves. *Vaccine* **2016**, *34*, 3051–3058. [CrossRef]
22. Nicholas, R.A.; Ayling, R.D.; Stipkovits, L.P. An experimental vaccine for calf pneumonia caused by *Mycoplasma bovis*: Clinical, cultural, serological and pathological findings. *Vaccine* **2002**, *20*, 3569–3575. [CrossRef]
23. Vähänikkilä, N.; Pohjanvirta, T.; Haapala, V.; Simojoki, H.; Soveri, T.; Browning, G.F.; Pelkonen, S.; Wawegama, N.K.; Autio, T. Characterisation of the course of *Mycoplasma bovis* infection in naturally infected dairy herds. *Vet. Microbiol.* **2019**, *231*, 107–115. [CrossRef] [PubMed]
24. Nicholas, R.A. Bovine mycoplasmosis: Silent and deadly. *Vet. Rec.* **2011**, *168*, 459–462. [CrossRef] [PubMed]
25. Technical Advisory Group (TAG) Report. 2019. Available online: https://www.mpi.govt.nz/dmsdocument/37754-report-of-the-mycoplasma-bovis-technical-advisory-group-tag-in-response-to-the-terms-of-reference-june-2019-18-october-2019 (accessed on 5 August 2020).
26. Timonen, A.A.E.; Autio, T.; Pohjanvirta, T.; Häkkinen, L.; Katholm, J.; Petersen, A.; Mõtus, K.; Kalmus, P. Dynamics of the within-herd prevalence of *Mycoplasma bovis* intramammary infection in endemically infected dairy herds. *Vet. Microbiol.* **2020**, *242*, 108608. [CrossRef] [PubMed]
27. Gille, L.; Evrard, J.; Callens, J.; Supré, K.; Grégoire, F.; Boyen, F.; Haesebrouck, F.; Deprez, P.; Pardon, B. The presence of *Mycoplasma bovis* in colostrum. *Vet. Res.* **2020**, *51*, 54. [CrossRef]
28. Passchyn, P.; Piepers, S.; De Meulemeester, L.; Boyen, F.; Haesebrouck, F.; De Vliegher, S. Between-herd prevalence of *Mycoplasma bovis* in bulk milk in Flanders, Belgium. *Res. Vet. Sci.* **2012**, *92*, 219–220. [CrossRef]
29. Stott, G.H.; Wiersma, F.; Menefee, B.E.; Radwanski, F.R. Influence of environment on passive immunity in calves. *J. Dairy Sci.* **1976**, *59*, 1306–1311. [CrossRef]
30. Alabdullah, H.; Schneider, C.; Fox, L. Effect of dexamethasone administration on shedding of *Mycoplasma bovis* in calves. In Proceedings of the Third International Symposium on Mastitis and Milk Quality, St. Louis, MO, USA, 22–24 September 2011.
31. Alabdullah, H.A.; Fox, L.K.; Gay, J.M.; Barrington, G.M.; Mealey, R.H. Effects of dexamethasone and *Mycoplasma bovis* on bovine neutrophil function *in vitro*. *Vet. Immunol. Immunopathol.* **2015**, *164*, 67–73. [CrossRef]
32. Ayling, R.D.; Bashiruddin, S.E.; Nicholas, R.A.J. *Mycoplasma* species and related organisms isolated from ruminants in Britain between 1990 and 2000. *Vet. Rec.* **2004**, *155*, 413–416. [CrossRef]

33. Gagea, M.I.; Bateman, K.G.; Shanahan, R.A.; van Dreumel, T.; McEwen, B.J.; Carman, S.; Archambault, M.; Caswell, J.L. Naturally occurring *Mycoplasma bovis*-associated pneumonia and polyarthritis in feedlot beef calves. *J. Vet. Diagn. Invest.* **2006**, *18*, 29–40. [CrossRef]
34. Ryan, M.J.; Wyand, D.S.; Hill, D.L.; Tourtellotte, M.E.; Yang, T.J. Morphologic changes following intraarticular inoculation of *Mycoplasma bovis* in calves. *Vet. Pathol.* **1983**, *20*, 472–487. [CrossRef]
35. Foster, A.P.; Naylor, R.D.; Howie, N.M.; Nicholas, R.A.; Ayling, R.D. *Mycoplasma bovis* and otitis in dairy calves in the United Kingdom. *Vet. J.* **2009**, *179*, 455–457. [CrossRef] [PubMed]
36. Ayling, R.; Nicholas, R.; Hogg, R.; Wessels, J.; Scholes, S.; Byrne, W.; Hill, M.; Moriarty, J.; O'Brien, T. *Mycoplasma bovis* isolated from brain tissue of calves. *Vet. Rec.* **2005**, *156*, 391–392. [CrossRef] [PubMed]
37. Kanci, A.; Wawegama, N.K.; Marenda, M.S.; Mansell, P.D.; Browning, G.F.; Markham, P.F. Reproduction of respiratory mycoplasmosis in calves by exposure to an aerosolised culture of *Mycoplasma bovis*. *Vet. Microbiol.* **2017**, *210*, 167–173. [CrossRef] [PubMed]
38. Jasper, D.E.; Al-Aubaidi, J.M.; Fabricant, J. Epidemiologic observations on mycoplasma mastitis. *Cornell Vet.* **1974**, *64*, 407–415.
39. Maunsell, F.P.; Woolums, A.R.; Francoz, D.; Rosenbush, R.F.; Step, D.L.; Wilson, D.J.; Janzen, E.D. *Mycoplasma bovis* infections in cattle. ACVIM Consensus Statement. *J. Vet. Intern. Med.* **2011**, *25*, 772–783. [CrossRef]
40. Lysnyansky, I.; Freed, M.; Rosales, R.S.; Mikula, I.; Khateb, N.; Gerchman, I.; van Straten, M.; Levisohn, S. An overview of *Mycoplasma bovis* mastitis in Israel (2004–2014). *Vet. J.* **2016**, *207*, 180–183. [CrossRef]
41. Hermeyer, K.; Peters, M.; Brügmann, M.; Jacobsen, B.; Hewicker-Trautwein, M. Demonstration of *Mycoplasma bovis* by immunohistochemistry and in situ hybridization in an aborted bovine fetus and neonatal calf. *J. Vet. Diagn. Invest.* **2012**, *24*, 364–369. [CrossRef]
42. Pfützner, H.; Sachse, K. *Mycoplasma bovis* as an agent of mastitis, pneumonia, arthritis and genital disorders in cattle. *Rev. Sci. Tech. Off. Int. Epiz.* **1996**, *15*, 1477–1494. [CrossRef]
43. Poumarat, F.; Longchambon, D.; Martel, J.L. Application of dot immunobinding on membrane filtration (MF dot) to the study of relationships within "M. mycoides cluster" and within "glucose and arginine-negative cluster" of ruminant mycoplasmas. *Vet. Microbiol.* **1992**, *32*, 375–390. [CrossRef]
44. Nicholas, R.A.J.; Baker, S.E. Recovery of mycoplasmas from animals. In *Mycoplasma Protocols*; Miles, R.J., Nicholas, R.A.J., Eds.; Humana Press: Totowa, NJ, USA, 1998; pp. 37–44.
45. Behera, S.; Rana, R.; Gupta, P.K.; Kumar, D.; Sonal; Rekha, V.; Arun, T.R.; Jena, D. Development of real-time PCR assay for the detection of *Mycoplasma bovis*. *Trop. Anim. Health Prod.* **2018**, *50*, 875–882. [CrossRef]
46. Andrés-Lasheras, S.; Zaheer, R.; Ha, R.; Lee, C.; Jelinski, M.; McAllister, T.A. A direct qPCR screening approach to improve the efficiency of *Mycoplasma bovis* isolation in the frame of a broad surveillance study. *J. Microbiol. Methods* **2020**, *169*, 105805. [CrossRef] [PubMed]
47. Appelt, S.; Aly, S.S.; Tonooka, K.; Glenn, K.; Xue, Z.; Lehenbauer, T.W.; Marco, M.L. Development and comparison of loop-mediated isothermal amplification and quantitative polymerase chain reaction assays for the detection of *Mycoplasma bovis* in milk. *J. Dairy Sci.* **2019**, *102*, 1985–1996. [CrossRef] [PubMed]
48. Parker, A.M.; House, J.K.; Hazelton, M.S.; Bosward, K.L.; Sheehy, P.A. Comparison of culture and a multiplex probe PCR for identifying *Mycoplasma* species in bovine milk, semen and swab samples. *PLoS ONE* **2017**, *12*, e0173422. [CrossRef] [PubMed]
49. Pansri, P.; Katholm, J.; Krogh, K.M.; Aagaard, A.K.; Schmidt, L.M.B.; Kudirkiene, E.; Larsen, L.E.; Olsen, J.E. Evaluation of novel multiplex qPCR assays for diagnosis of pathogens associated with the bovine respiratory disease complex. *Vet. J.* **2020**, *256*, 105425. [CrossRef] [PubMed]
50. Conrad, C.C.; Daher, R.K.; Stanford, K.; Amoako, K.K.; Boissinot, M.; Bergeron, M.G.; Alexander, T.; Cook, S.; Ralston, B.; Zaheer, R.; et al. A Sensitive and Accurate Recombinase Polymerase Amplification Assay for Detection of the Primary Bacterial Pathogens Causing Bovine Respiratory Disease. *Front. Vet. Sci.* **2020**, *7*, 208. [CrossRef] [PubMed]
51. Ashraf, A.; Imran, M.; Yaqub, T.; Tayyab, M.; Shehzad, W.; Mingala, C.N.; Chang, Y.-F. Development and validation of a loop-mediated isothermal amplification assay for the detection of *Mycoplasma bovis* in mastitic milk. *Folia Microb.* **2018**, *63*, 373–380. [CrossRef]
52. Itoh, M.; Hirano, Y.; Yamakawa, K.; Yasutomi, I.; Kuramoto, K.; Furuok, M.; Yamada, K. Combination of procedure for ultra rapid extraction (PURE) and loop-mediated isothermal amplification (LAMP) for rapid detection of *Mycoplasma bovis* in milk. *J. Vet. Med. Sci.* **2020**, 19–0695. [CrossRef]

53. Zhao, G.; Hou, P.; Huan, Y.; He, C.; Wang, H.; He, H. Development of a recombinase polymerase amplification combined with a lateral flow dipstick assay for rapid detection of the *Mycoplasma bovis*. *BMC Vet. Res.* **2018**, *14*, 412. [CrossRef]
54. Bokma, J.; Van Driessche, L.; Deprez, P.; Haesebrouck, F.; Vahl, M.; Weesendorp, E.; Deurenberg, R.H.; Pardon, P.; Boyen, P. Rapid identification of 1 *Mycoplasma bovis* from bovine bronchoalveolar lavage fluid with MALDI-TOF MS after enrichment procedure. *J. Clin. Microbiol.* **2020**, *58*, e00004-20. [CrossRef]
55. Thurmond, M.C.; Tyler, J.W.; Luiz, D.M.; Holmberg, C.A.; Picanso, J.P. The effect of pre-enrichment on recovery of *Streptococcus agalactiae*, *Staphylococcus aureus* and mycoplasma from bovine milk. *Epidemiol. Infect.* **1989**, *103*, 465–474. [CrossRef]
56. Punyapornwithaya, V.; Fox, L.K.; Gay, G.M.; Hancock, D.D.; Alldredge, J.R. Short communication: The effect of centrifugation and resuspension on the recovery of *Mycoplasma species* from milk. *J. Dairy Sci.* **2009**, *92*, 4444–4447. [CrossRef] [PubMed]
57. Li, Y.; Fan, P.; Zhou, S.; Zhang, L. Loop-mediated isothermal amplification (LAMP): A novel rapid detection platform for pathogens. *Microb. Pathog.* **2017**, *107*, 54–61. [CrossRef] [PubMed]
58. Nunoya, T.; Omori, T.; Tomioka, H.; Umeda, F.; Suzuki, T.; Uetsuka, K. Intracellular Localization of Mycoplasma bovis in the Bronchiolar Epithelium of Experimentally Infected Calves. *J. Comp. Path.* **2020**, *176*, 14–18. [CrossRef] [PubMed]
59. Kleinschmidt, S.; Spergser, J.; Rosengarten, R.; Hewicker-Trautwein, M. Long-term survival of *Mycoplasma bovis* in necrotic lesions and in phagocytic cells as demonstrated by transmission and immunogold electron microscopy in lung tissue from experimentally infected calves. *Vet. Microbiol.* **2013**, *162*, 949–953. [CrossRef] [PubMed]
60. Bell-Rogers, P.; Parker, L.; Cai, H.Y. Multi-locus sequence types of *Mycoplasma bovis* isolated from Ontario, Canada in the past three decades have a temporal distribution. *J. Vet. Diagn. Invest.* **2018**, *30*, 130–135. [CrossRef]
61. Register, K.B.; Lysnyansky, I.; Jelinski, M.D.; Boatwright, W.D.; Waldner, M.; Bayles, D.O.; Pilo, P.; Alt, D.P. Comparison of two multilocus sequence typing schemes for *Mycoplasma bovis* and revision of the PubMLST reference method. *J. Clin. Microbiol.* **2020**, *58*, e00283-20. [CrossRef]
62. Yair, Y.; Borovok, I.; Mikula, I.; Falk, R.; Fox, L.K.; Gophna, U.; Lysnyansky, I. Genomics-based epidemiology of bovine *Mycoplasma bovis* strains in Israel. *BMC Genom.* **2020**, *21*, 70. [CrossRef]
63. Parker, A.M.; Shukla, A.; House, J.K.; Hazelton, M.S.; Bosward, K.L.; Kokotovic, B.; Sheehy, P.A. Genetic characterization of Australian *Mycoplasma bovis* isolates through whole genome sequencing analysis. *Vet. Microbiol.* **2016**, *196I*, 118–125. [CrossRef]
64. Rasheed, M.A.; Qi, J.; Zhu, X.; Chenfei, H.; Menghwar, H.; Khan, F.A.; Guo, A. Comparative genomics of *Mycoplasma bovis* strains reveals that decreased virulence with increasing passages might correlate with potential virulence-related factors. *Front. Cell. Infect. Microbiol.* **2017**, *7*, 177. [CrossRef]
65. Sachse, K.; Pfützner, H.; Hötzel, H.; Demuth, B.; Heller, M.; Berthold, E. Comparison of various diagnostic methods for the detection of *Mycoplasma bovis*. *Rev. Sci. Tech.-Off. Int. Epiz.* **1993**, *12*, 571–580. [CrossRef]
66. Nielsen, P.K.; Petersen, M.B.; Nielsen, L.R.; Halasa, T.; Toft, N. Latent class analysis of bulk tank milk PCR and ELISA testing for herd level diagnosis of *Mycoplasma bovis*. *Prev. Vet. Med.* **2015**, *121*, 338–342. [CrossRef] [PubMed]
67. Gille, L.; Callens, J.; Supré, K.; Boyen, F.; Haesebrouck, F.; Van Driessche, L.; van Leenen, K.; Deprez, P.; Pardon, B. Use of breeding bull and absence of a calving pen as a risk factors for the presence of *Mycoplasma bovis* in dairy herds. *J. Dairy Sci.* **2018**, *101*, 8284–8290. [CrossRef] [PubMed]
68. Andersson, A.-M.; Aspán, A.; Wisselink, H.J.; Smid, B.; Ridley, A.; Pelkonen, S.; Autio, T.; Lauritsen, K.T.; Kensø, J.; Gaurivaud, P.; et al. A European inter-laboratory trial to evaluate the performance of three serological methods for diagnosis of *Mycoplasma bovis* infection in cattle using latent class analysis. *BMC Vet. Res.* **2019**, *15*, 369. [CrossRef] [PubMed]
69. Wawegama, N.K.; Browning, G.F.; Kanci, A.; Marenda, M.S.; Markham, F.F. Development of a Recombinant Protein-Based Enzyme-Linked Immunosorbent Assay for Diagnosis of *Mycoplasma bovis* Infection in Cattle. *Clin. Vaccine Immunol.* **2014**, *21*, 196–202. [CrossRef] [PubMed]
70. Petersen, M.B.; Wawegama, N.K.; Denwood, M.; Markham, P.F.; Browning, G.F.; Nielsen, L.R. *Mycoplasma bovis* antibody dynamics in naturally exposed dairy calves according to two diagnostic tests. *BMC Vet. Res.* **2018**, *14*, 258. [CrossRef] [PubMed]

71. Wisselink, H.J.; Smid, B.; Plater, J.; Ridley, A.; Andersson, A.-M.; Aspán, A.; Pohjanvirta, T.; Vähänikkilä, N.; Larsen, H.; Høgberg, J.; et al. A European interlaboratory trial to evaluate the performance of different PCR methods for *Mycoplasma bovis* diagnosis. *BMC Vet. Res.* **2019**, *15*, 86. [CrossRef]
72. Chazel, M.; Tardy, F.; Le Grand, D.; Calavas, D.; Poumarat, F. Mycoplasmoses of ruminants in France: Recent data from the national surveillance network. *BMC Vet. Res.* **2010**, *6*, 32. [CrossRef]
73. Mackie, D.P.; Finley, D.; Brice, N.; Ball, H.J. Mixed mycoplasma mastitis outbreak in a dairy herd. *Vet. Rec.* **2000**, *147*, 335–336. [CrossRef]
74. Jasper, D.E. Prevalence of mycoplasmal mastitis in the western states. *Calif. Vet.* **1980**, *43*, 24–26.
75. McAuliffe, L.; Ellis, R.J.; Lawes, J.R.; Ayling, R.D.; Nicholas, R.A.J. 16S rDNA PCR and denaturing gradient gel electrophoresis; a single generic test for detecting and differentiating *Mycoplasma* species. *J. Med. Microbiol.* **2005**, *54*, 731–739. [CrossRef]
76. Loy, J.D.; Leger, L.; Workman, A.M.; Clawson, M.L.; Bulut, E.; Wang, B. Development of a multiplex real-time PCR assay using two thermocycling platforms for detection of major bacterial pathogens associated with bovine respiratory disease complex from clinical samples. *J. Vet. Diagn. Invest.* **2018**, *30*, 837–847. [CrossRef] [PubMed]
77. Pereyre, S.; Tardy, F.; Renaudin, H.; Cauvin, E.; Del Prá Netto Machado, L.; Tricot, A.; Benoit, F.; Treilles, M.; Bébéar, C. Identification and Subtyping of Clinically Relevant Human and Ruminant Mycoplasmas by Use of Matrix-Assisted Laser Desorption Ionization–Time of Flight Mass Spectrometry *J. Clin. Microbiol.* **2013**, *51*, 3314–3323. [CrossRef] [PubMed]
78. O'Farrell, K.; Dillon, P.; Mee, j.; Crosse, S.; Nnolan, M.; Byrne, N.; Reidy, M.; Flynn, F.; Condon, T. Strategy for restocking Moorepark after depopulation following BSE. *Ir. Vet. J.* **2001**, *54*, 70–75.
79. Lysnyansky, I.; Mikula, I.; Ozeri, R.; Bellaiche, M.; Nicholas, R.A.J.; van Straten, M. Mycoplasma bovis Seroprevalence in Israeli Dairy Herds, Feedlots and Imported Cattle. *Isr. J. Vet. Med.* **2017**, *72*, 13–16.
80. Stabel, J.R.; Hurd, S.; Calvente, L.; Rosenbusch, R.F. Destruction of *Mycobacterium paratuberculosis, Salmonella* spp., and *Mycoplasma* spp. in raw milk by a commercial on-farm high-temperature, short-time pasteurizer. *J. Dairy Sci.* **2004**, *87*, 2177–2183. [CrossRef]
81. Gelsinger, S.L.; Heinrichs, A.J. Comparison of immune responses in calves fed heat-treated or unheated colostrum. *J. Dairy Sci.* **2017**, *100*, 4090–4101. [CrossRef] [PubMed]
82. Higuchi, H.; Gondaira, S.; Iwano, H.; Hirose, K.; Nakajima, K.; Kawai, K.; Hagiwara, K.; Tamura, Y.; Nagahata, H. *Mycoplasma* species isolated from intramammary infection of Japanese dairy cows. *Vet. Rec.* **2013**, *172*, 557. [CrossRef]
83. Kauf, A.C.; Rosenbusch, R.F.; Paape, M.J.; Bannerman, D.D. Innate immune response to intramammary *Mycoplasma bovis* infection. *J. Dairy Sci.* **2007**, *90*, 3336–3348. [CrossRef]
84. Punyapornwithaya, V.; Fox, L.K.; Hancock, D.D.; Gay, J.M.; Wenz, J.R.; Alldredge, J.R. Incidence and transmission of *Mycoplasma bovis* mastitis in Holstein dairy cows in a hospital pen: A case study. *Prev. Vet. Med.* **2011**, *98*, 74–78. [CrossRef]
85. Murai, K.; Lehenbauer, T.W.; Champagne, J.D.; Glenn, K.; Aly, S.S. Cost-effectiveness of diagnostic strategies using quantitative real-time PCR and bacterial culture to identify contagious mastitis cases in large dairy herds. *Prev. Vet. Med.* **2014**, *113*, 522–535. [CrossRef]
86. Mahdizadeh, S.; Sawford, K.; van Andel, M.; Browning, G.F. Efficacy of citric acid and sodium hypochlorite as disinfectants against *Mycoplasma bovis*. *Vet. Microbiol.* **2020**, *243*, 108630. [CrossRef] [PubMed]
87. Boddie, R.L.; Owens, W.E.; Ray, C.H.; Nickerson, S.C.; Boddie, N.T. Germicidal activities of representatives of five different teat dip classes against three bovine mycoplasma species using a modified excised teat model. *J. Dairy Sci.* **2002**, *85*, 1909–1912. [CrossRef]

pathogens

MDPI

Article

Analysis of the Leukocyte Response in Calves Suffered from *Mycoplasma bovis* Pneumonia

Katarzyna Dudek [1,*], Dariusz Bednarek [1], Urszula Lisiecka [2], Anna Kycko [3], Michał Reichert [3], Krzysztof Kostro [2,†] and Stanisław Winiarczyk [2]

1 Department of Cattle and Sheep Diseases, National Veterinary Research Institute, 57 Partyzantów Avenue, 24-100 Pulawy, Poland; dbednarek@piwet.pulawy.pl
2 Department of Epizootiology and Clinic of Infectious Diseases, Faculty of Veterinary Medicine, University of Life Sciences in Lublin, 30 Głęboka Street, 20-612 Lublin, Poland; urszula.lisiecka@up.lublin.pl (U.L.); genp53@interia.pl (S.W.)
3 Department of Pathology, National Veterinary Research Institute, 57 Partyzantów Avenue, 24-100 Pulawy, Poland; anna.kycko@piwet.pulawy.pl (A.K.); reichert@piwet.pulawy.pl (M.R.)
* Correspondence: katarzyna.dudek@piwet.pulawy.pl
† This author has passed away in 2018.

Received: 29 April 2020; Accepted: 22 May 2020; Published: 24 May 2020

Abstract: *Mycoplasma bovis* is known to be a cause of chronic pneumonia in cattle. To date, the disease pathomechanism has not been fully elucidated. Leukocytes play a key role in host antimicrobial defense mechanisms. Many in vitro studies of the effect of *Mycoplasma bovis* (*M. bovis*) on leukocytes have been performed, but it is difficult to apply these results to in vivo conditions. Additionally, only a few studies on a local immune response in *M. bovis* pneumonia have been undertaken. In this study, the experimental calf-infection model was used to determine the effect of field *M. bovis* strains on changes of the peripheral blood leukocyte response, including phagocytic activity and oxygen metabolism by cytometry analyses. An additional aim was to evaluate the lung local immunity of the experimentally infected calves using immunohistochemical staining. The general stimulation of phagocytic and killing activity of peripheral blood leukocytes in response to the *M. bovis* infection points to upregulation of cellular antimicrobial mechanisms. The local immune response in the infected lungs was characterized by the T- and B-cell stimulation, however, most seen in the increased T lymphocyte response. Post-infection, strong expression of the antigen-presenting cells and phagocytes also confirmed the activation of lung local immunity. In this study—despite the stimulation—both the peripheral and local cellular antimicrobial mechanisms seem to appear ineffective in eliminating *M. bovis* from the host and preventing the specific lung lesions, indicating an ability of the pathogen to avoid the host immune response in the *M. bovis* pneumonia.

Keywords: *Mycoplasma bovis*; cattle; leukocytes; phagocytosis; oxygen metabolism

1. Introduction

Mycoplasma bovis causes many disorders in cattle, such as pneumonia, arthritis, mastitis and keratoconjunctivitis, from which chronic pneumonia is one of the most diagnosed [1–3]. To date, the pathomechanism of *M. bovis* pneumonia has not been fully elucidated. One such mechanism is the ability of the pathogen to modulate the host immune response [4]. It has been previously confirmed that *M. bovis* possesses both immunostimulating and immunosuppressive properties, most demonstrated in vitro studies. *M. bovis* can induce strong TNF-α responses in the exposed macrophages isolated from mycoplasma-free bronchoalveolar lavages of adult cattle [5]. The ability of *M. bovis* to modulate different neutrophil functions has been demonstrated by Jimbo et al. [6]. After incubation of *M. bovis* with neutrophils isolated from clinically healthy animals the induction of the cell apoptosis and increased elastase production was observed. The same study showed upregulation of pro-inflammatory cytokines—i.e., TNF-α and IL-12—but with no effect on TGF-β production [6]. Otherwise, it was revealed that *M. bovis* can inhibit the oxygen-dependent microbicidal response of neutrophils isolated from the peripheral blood of adult cattle [7]. In vitro conditions, *M. bovis* is also able to suppress a phytohemagglutinin-induced stimulation of bovine peripheral blood lymphocytes, however with no cytotoxic effect [8]. Similarly, other in vitro study demonstrated the ability of *M. bovis* to inhibit a Concanavalin A-induced proliferation of peripheral blood lymphocytes isolated from *M. bovis* negative donor cattle [9]. Despite so many results, the data received is still not endless, especially since it is not often possible to interpret in vitro results for in vivo conditions. Additionally, only a few studies on the characterization of the local immune response in *M. bovis* pneumonia in calves were undertaken [10,11].

To better advance our knowledge of the disease pathomechanism, an in vivo study using the experimental animal model on calves was performed which evaluated the effect of *M. bovis* on bovine peripheral blood leukocytes. To better control the *M. bovis* infection, an additional aim was to evaluate the lung local immunity of calves experimentally infected with the pathogen.

2. Results

Infection efficacy in the experimental calves was confirmed by clinical, post mortem and histopathologic observations and the results of immunohistochemistry (IHC) and enzyme-linked immunosorbent assay (ELISA) analyses for *M. bovis* antigen were described previously by Dudek et al. [12]. Following the calf infection with *M. bovis*, extensive caseous necrosis and lobular consolidation were observed. The *M. bovis* antigen was detected in epithelial cells of bronchioli in the lungs of all experimental calves as opposed to the controls, which were negative. All detailed post mortem results were previously described by Dudek et al. [12].

2.1. Hematology

Following infection, the white blood cell (WBC) count was generally comparable to the control group throughout the study, with no significant differences ($p < 0.05$). However, the analysis of leucogram showed a comparable or lower percentage of the lymphocytes (LYM) in the experimental group throughout the study compared to the control group, with significantly lower values on Day 3 post the first infecting dose. In the experimental group, the monocyte (MON) percentage did not differ significantly ($p < 0.05$) from the control group throughout the study. However, the granulocyte (GRA) percentage was increased post the infection throughout the study compared to the control group and reached significantly ($p < 0.05$) higher values than the control group on Day 3 post the first infecting dose (Figure 1). Numerical values are presented in Figure S1.

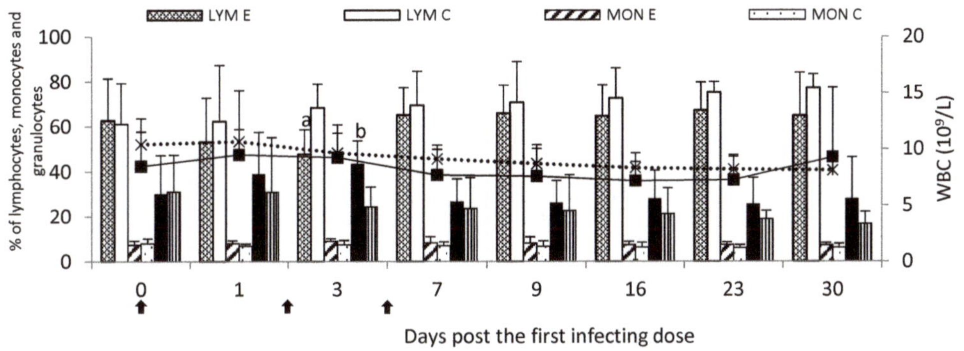

Figure 1. WBC count and a mean percentage of granulocytes, monocytes and lymphocytes in the peripheral blood of calves following infection with *M. bovis*. E—experimental group; C—control group; ⬆—single infecting dose of *M. bovis*; a—$p < 0.05$ between the experimental and control groups for lymphocytes; b—$p < 0.05$ between the experimental and control groups for granulocytes.

2.2. Flow Cytometry

2.2.1. Lymphocyte Phenotyping

There were no significant ($p < 0.05$) differences between the experimental and control groups in the percentage of $CD2^+$, $CD4^+$ and $CD8^+$ cells throughout the study. However, on Day 3 post the first infecting dose, the $CD4^+$ percentage was significantly lower ($p \leq 0.05$) than the control group (Figure 2). Numerical values were presented in Supplementary Figure S2.

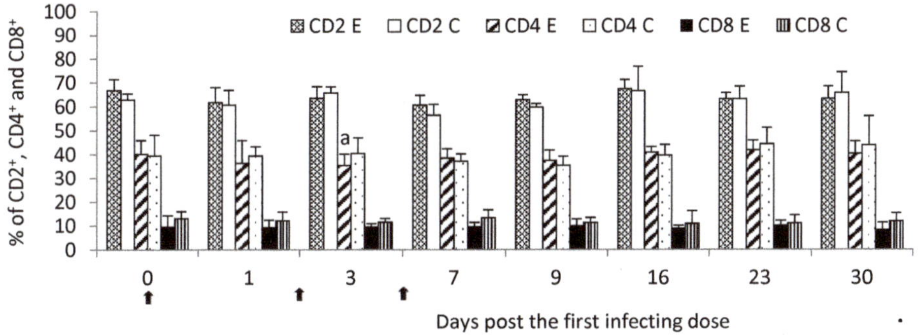

Figure 2. $CD2^+$, $CD4^+$ and $CD8^+$ mean percentage in the peripheral blood of calves following infection with *M. bovis*. E—experimental group; C—control group. ⬆—single infecting dose of *M. bovis*; a—$p < 0.05$ between the experimental and control groups for $CD4^+$.

2.2.2. Phagocytic Activity and Oxygen Metabolism of Leukocytes

The percentage of phagocytic granulocytes in the peripheral blood of the experimental group did not significantly differ ($p < 0.05$) from the control group throughout the study. However, the mean fluorescence intensity (MFI) for granulocytes visibly increased on Day 9 post the first infecting dose and it was statistically significantly higher ($p < 0.05$) than the control group on Day 16 (Figure 3). Numerical values were presented in Figure S3.

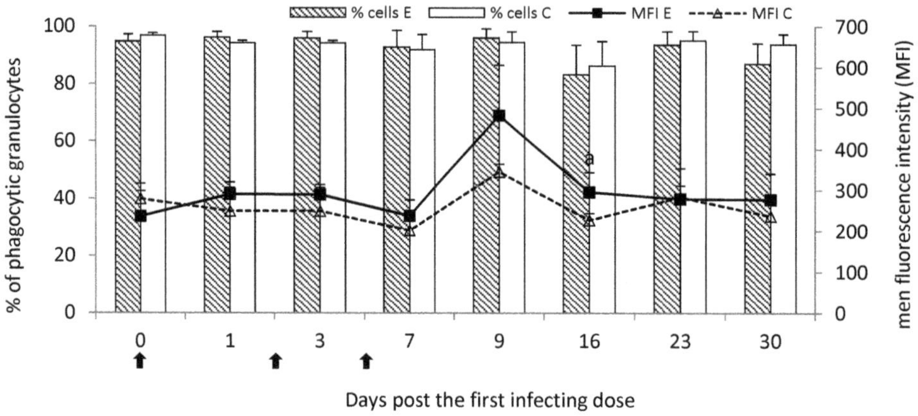

Figure 3. Phagocytic activity of granulocytes in the peripheral blood of calves following infection with *M. bovis* expressed as a mean percentage of phagocytic cells (bar graph) and mean fluorescence intensity (MFI; linear graph). E—experimental group; C—control group. 🠉—single infecting dose of *M. bovis*; a—$p < 0.05$ between the experimental and control groups for MFI.

Following the infection, the percentage of phagocytic monocytes was generally comparable to the control group throughout the study, with the exception of Day 9, when lower values were observed. However, on Day 23, a visible increase in the percentage in the experimental group was observed. Following the infection, the MFI for monocytes was generally slightly higher than the control group throughout the study, especially on Day one following the first infecting dose. However, no significant differences ($p < 0.05$) between the experimental and control groups on the phagocytic cell percentage and MFI were observed (Figure 4). Numerical values were presented in Figure S4.

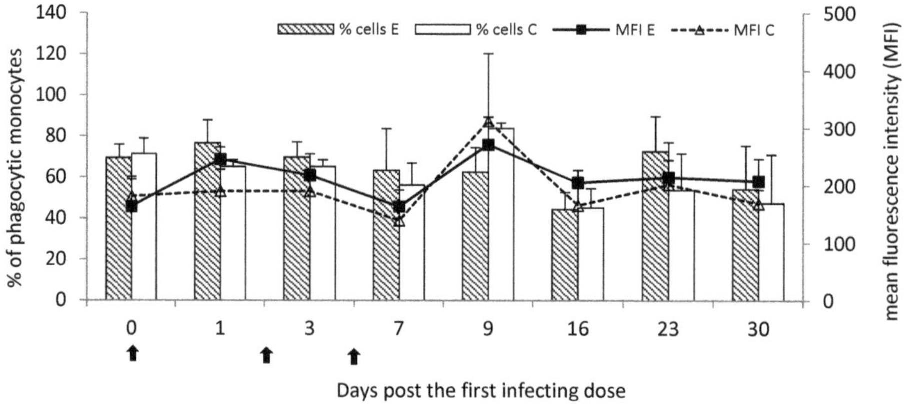

Figure 4. The phagocytic activity of monocytes in the peripheral blood of calves following infection with *M. bovis* expressed as a mean percentage of phagocytic cells (bar graph) and mean fluorescence intensity (MFI; linear graph). E—experimental group; C—control group. 🠉—single infecting dose of *M. bovis*.

For the oxygen metabolism, the percentage of activated leukocytes was significantly increased ($p < 0.05$) on Day one post the first infecting dose, however after that it suddenly decreased and had similar or lower values than the control group until the end of the study with significantly lower values ($p < 0.05$) on Day 23. The MFI was generally increased in the experimental group throughout the study when compared to the control group, however with no significant ($p < 0.05$) differences (Figure 5). Numerical values were presented in Figure S5.

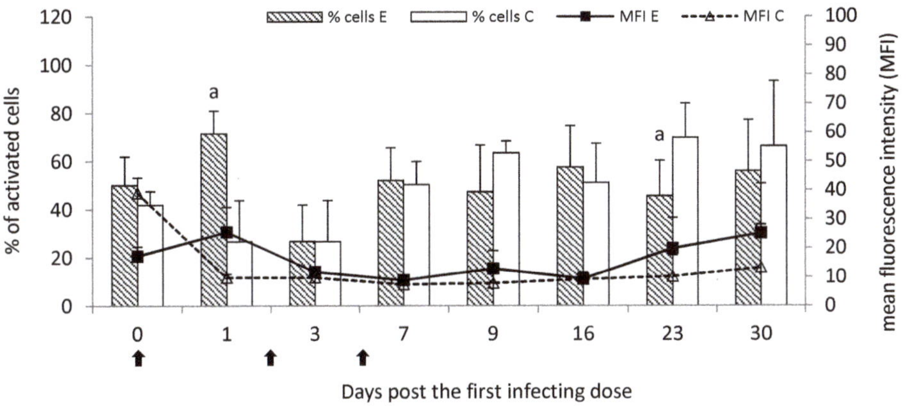

Figure 5. Oxygen metabolism of leukocytes in peripheral blood of calves following infection with *M. bovis* expressed as a mean percentage of cells (bar graph) and mean fluorescence intensity (MFI; linear graph) after activation by *E. coli*. E—experimental group; C—control group. ⬆—single infecting dose of *M. bovis*. a—$p < 0.05$ between the experimental and control groups for percentage of cells.

2.3. Immunohistochemistry

In the lungs of experimentally infected calves, multiple foci of CD3 positive cells were visible in the lung parenchyma, within the hyperplastic bronchus-associated lymphoid tissue (BALT) and peribronchiolar infiltrations (Figure 6A). In the control calves, the positive reaction for the CD3 antigen was visible in BALT (Figure 6B). The positive labeling for CD79a in the infected calves was present in the hyperplastic BALT and, to a lesser extent, in the cells around bronchioli or the cells infiltrating necrotic areas (Figure 6C). In the control animals, the reaction for the CD79a antigen was visible in BALT (Figure 6D). As a result of CD3 and CD79a quantification, the immunopositive cell counts determined as mean value ± standard deviation (SD) in the control group were 1408.8 ± 88.1 for CD3 and 1437.5 ± 267 for CD79a. In the experimental group the mean cell counts for CD3 and CD79a were 3823.7 ± 1551.3 and 2118.7 ± 730.18, respectively. Compared to the controls, the experimental group displayed a significant increase ($p < 0.05$) in the number of both CD3- and CD79a-positive cells, however within the group, the mean cell count value was significantly higher ($p < 0.05$) for CD3 than for CD79a.

In the lungs of the experimentally infected calves, the high concentration of MHC class II marker was found in the lymphoid cells infiltrating the granulomas, in BALT as well as in bronchiolar epithelium and the lymphoid cells in the alveolar walls (Figure 7A), while in the control animals the positive labeling for MHC class II was seen in BALT, the epithelial cells of bronchioli and in some lymphoid cells within the lung parenchyma (Figure 7B). When assessing the presence of S100 marker in the lungs of the infected calves, its high concentration was observed in vascular endothelial cells, as well as in some cells forming cellular infiltrates within granulomas (Figure 7C). In the control group, the positive IHC response was only demonstrated in vascular endothelial cells (Figure 7D).

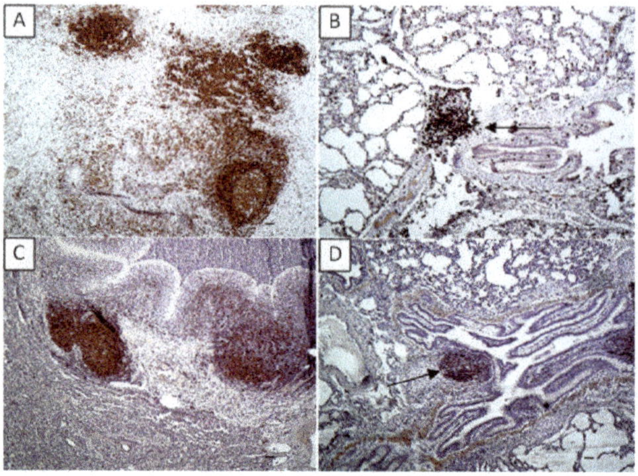

Figure 6. The lungs of the calves experimentally infected with *Mycoplasma bovis* (**A**,**C**), lungs of the control calves (**B**,**D**), IHC. (**A**) lung of an experimental calf. Positive immunolabeling of CD3 visible as dark brown staining in the hyperplastic bronchus-associated lymphoid tissue (BALT) and lymphoid cells scattered in the lung parenchyma. Bar = 50 μm; (**B**) lung of control calf. Positive immunolabeling of CD3 visible in BALT (arrow) and the single cells scattered in the lung parenchyma. Bar = 50 μm; (**C**) lung of an experimental calf. Positive immunolabeling of CD79a visible as dark brown staining in the hyperplastic BALT and lymphoid cells scattered in the lung parenchyma. Bar = 50 μm; (**D**) lung of control calf. Positive immunolabeling of CD79a visible in BALT (arrow). Bar = 50 μm.

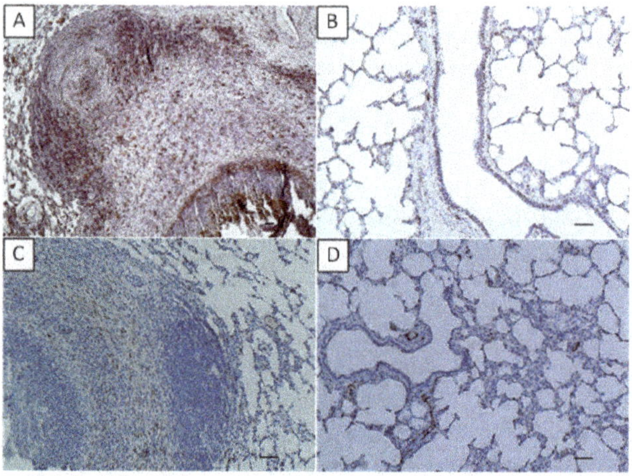

Figure 7. The lungs of the calves experimentally infected with *Mycoplasma bovis* (**A**,**C**), the lungs of the control calves (**B**,**D**), IHC. (**A**) lung of an experimental calf. Positive labeling of MHC class II visible as the brown staining in BALT, in the cells within the infiltrates surrounding the necrotic masses (right bottom) and in the single cells scattered in the lung parenchyma (left side). Bar = 50 μm (**B**) lung of control calf. Positive labeling of MHC class II visible as brown staining in the bronchiolar epithelial layer and the single cells around the bronchus. Bar = 50 μm; (**C**) lung of an experimental calf. Positive labeling of S100 visible as the brown staining in several cells within the granuloma. Bar = 50 μm; (**D**) lung of control calf. Positive labeling of S100 is visible in the endothelium of the blood capillaries. Bar = 50 μm.

3. Discussion

In the current study, the lung local immune response to *M. bovis* infection was characterized by the lymphocyte stimulation dependent on both the T- and B-cell responses, however, the most seen in the strong immunohistochemical labeling of T lymphocytes. It had a reflection in a general decrease in the percent of circulating lymphocytes, the most intensified post the second infecting dose of *M. bovis*. It was additionally confirmed by flow cytometry analysis which showed at the same time point a decline in the T-helper cell percentage. It was probably due to the migration of the lymphocytes from peripheral blood to sites of infection, including lung tissue. At the same point in time post the infection, a decrease in the percentage of circulating lymphocytes was compensated by the increased percentage of other leukocyte populations like granulocytes possibly indicating an enhancement production of these cells in the bone marrow and their release into the peripheral blood. Hermeyer et al. [11] examined the expression of CD3, CD79a, S100A8 and S100A9 markers within the lungs of the aborted bovine fetus and the newborn calf died with severe respiratory symptoms, both suffered from suppurative bronchointerstitial pneumonia due to *M. bovis* infection. The results of the study indicated the increased lymphocytic aggregates expressed CD3 and CD79a within the lung tissues of both animals confirming the presence of both T and B lymphocytes. All this suggests the activation of specific local immunity to *M. bovis* lung infection as was confirmed in the current study [11]. In another study, the identification and quantitative evaluation of $CD4^{+}$ and $CD8^{+}$ T lymphocytes using IHC staining in the chronic *M. bovis* pneumonia was performed. However, post the experimental infection of calves with *M. bovis*, no significant differences in the numbers of both cells in BALT of bronchioli were observed compared to the control [10].

Neutrophils and macrophages are known to be important in innate immune mechanisms in the lung, including bacteria recognizing and phagocytosis needed for the antigen presentation [4]. In the study of Hermeyer et al. [11], the increased number of macrophages expressed both S100A8 and S100A9 in the lung parenchyma of the aborted bovine fetus and neonatal calf affected with *M. bovis* was shown. Additionally, within the lung of aborted bovine fetus neutrophilic aggregates were presented [11]. In our *M. bovis* calf-infection model the increased S100 expression in the infected lungs was observed probably indicating the stimulation of phagocyte response according to Hermeyer et al. [11]. As previously proved, there is a phenomenon of *M. bovis* surviving nearby necrosis areas despite the presence of a large number of infiltrating cells like neutrophils and macrophages [13,14].

In the study of Hermeyer et al. [10] in the lungs of *M. bovis*-infected calves' immunoreactivity of MHC class II varied dependent on the affected area. The strong MHC class II expression was revealed on the lymphoid cells in hyperplastic BALT, whereas the weak immunoreactivity or negative reaction was observed in intra-alveolar as well as perinecrotic located macrophages and in areas near caseonecrotic lesions. According to the author, such location of MHC class II expression suggest on one hand, ongoing stimulation of the lung local immunity and on the other hand downregulation of the antigen-presenting mechanisms in chronic *M. bovis* pneumonia [10]. In the current study, the high concentration of MHC class II was found in both the BALT and within the infiltrates surrounding the necrotic masses indicating general upregulation of the antigen-presenting mechanisms in response to the *M. bovis* infection. All this seems to confirm the formation of antigen-MHC class II complexes in the infected lungs, their recognition by the activated T lymphocytes and further activation of B-cell dependent response to generate specific immunity.

It is well known that granulocytes—especially neutrophils—are crucial cells in host antimicrobial defense [15]. As a predominant population of circulating leukocytes, neutrophils play an important role in the first line of cellular defense of the host against invading pathogens by various functions, including phagocytosis and oxidative burst [6,16]. In the current study, the percentage of circulating granulocytes was increased post *M. bovis* infection. It had a reflection in the slight increase in the percentage of phagocytic granulocytes at the initial stage of the disease. As the disease progresses, the visible drop in the percentage of phagocytic cells was observed, the most seen at the end of the study (a chronic stage of the disease). However, the number of phagocytosed bacteria by granulocytes on Day

16 post the first infecting dose of *M. bovis* was significantly higher than the control despite the beginning of the decline in the percentage of phagocytic cells possibly indicating increased antimicrobial activity of the cells.

Marked, however not statistically significant stimulation of phagocytic activity at the most time points post the infection was observed for circulating monocytes. Unlike granulocytes, the percentage of phagocytic monocytes was visibly increased at the chronic stage of the disease.

In the current study, the analysis of oxygen metabolism of peripheral blood leukocytes showed the initial increase in the percentage of the activated cells to different extents, the most seen post the first infecting dose of *M. bovis*. It was reflected in the visibly increased killing activity of these cells. In turn, a further decline in the activated cell percentage probably resulted from the subsequent doses of *M. bovis* and the chronic stage of the disease. It was probably in favor of mobilizing these cells within the lungs against the persisting/survival of *M. bovis* antigen. However, the killing activity of circulating leukocytes at that time was enhanced, despite the decrease in the percentage of the activated cells, possibly indicating releasing of *M. bovis* from sites of the infection, including lung tissue. In the study of Wiggins et al. [17], the effect of multiple *M. bovis* isolates (field, clinical and high passage laboratory) on Reactive Oxygen Species (ROS) production by blood leukocytes isolated from six cattle using an oxidation of dihydrorhodamine 123 (DHR-123) was measured. The leukocyte incubation with both field and clinical *M. bovis* isolates generally impaired ROS production, as opposed to the laboratory ones. In this study, the leukocyte metabolic activity using the reduction of 3-(4,5-dimethylthiazol-2-yl)-2,5-diphenyltetrazolium bromide (MTT) was also determined. Mostly following the exposure to all *M. bovis* isolates no effect on cellular metabolism of the bovine leukocytes was shown, indicating that observed suppression of ROS generation was not dependent on the leukocyte impairment of metabolic functions [17].

In the current study, using the *M. bovis* calf-infection model, the changes in the phagocytic activity and oxygen-dependent killing in the peripheral blood leukocytes was related to the stage of *M. bovis* pneumonia. However, the general stimulation of phagocytic and killing activity of circulating leukocytes in response to the *M. bovis* infection points to the upregulation of cellular antimicrobial mechanisms. The general depletion in the percent of circulating lymphocytes supporting the ongoing infection with *M. bovis*. The lung local immune response to the *M. bovis* experimental infection was characterized by the lymphocyte stimulation, the most seen in the increased T-cell response. The calf infection with *M. bovis* also caused the increased expression of the antigen-presenting cells, as well as the phagocytes further confirming the activation of lung local immune response. Despite the general stimulation of both peripheral and local cellular antimicrobial mechanisms, their effectiveness appeared insufficient in eliminating the bacteria from the host and preventing specific *M. bovis* lesions, indicating the ability of the bacteria to avoid the host immune response in *M. bovis* pneumonia.

4. Materials and Methods

4.1. Animals

Experimental study on animals was carried out in accordance with the requirements of the Local Ethics Committee on Animal Experimentation of the University of Life Sciences in Lublin, Poland (Decision no. 102/2015 admitted 8 Dec 2015), which also meet the EU standards.

The study was performed on 10 four-week-old, clinically healthy female calves housed in the institute's vivarium. Before the proper study, the nasal swabs and blood samples were collected from the calves and examined for *Mycoplasma bovis* and other respiratory pathogens detection which was described previously by Dudek et al. [12]. After a three-week adaptive period, the calves were divided into two groups: experimental (n = 6) and control (n = 4).

All detailed information about the animals and methods used for confirmation of the infection efficacy was described previously by Dudek et al. [12].

4.2. Calf Challenge

The experimental calves were three times infected with 23 mL of inoculum containing the field *M. bovis* strain KP795974 suspended in sterile phosphate-buffered saline pH 7.2 (PBS), with a concentration of 1.5×10^8 CFU/mL. The inoculum was prepared as described previously [18] and given three times in total; for the first time on Day 0 of the study and then two times at 48 h intervals; twice intratracheally and once by a nasal aerosol application. Instead, the control animals were administered with sterile PBS. It was described previously in detail by Dudek et al. [12].

4.3. Sample Collection

Blood samples were collected in EDTA tubes (for hematology and CD marker detection) or standard heparinized tubes (concerning analyses of phagocytic activity and oxygen metabolism of leukocytes) on Days 0, 1, 3, 7, 9, 16, 23 and 30 post the first *M. bovis* infecting dose. At the end of the experiment on Day 30, all experimental and two control calves were euthanized to collect the lung samples for pathologic and immunohistochemical analyses.

4.4. Hematology

White blood cell (WBC) count and percentage of lymphocytes, monocytes and granulocytes were calculated in an automatic veterinary blood analyzer (Exigo, Boule Medical AB, Spånga, Sweden).

4.5. Flow Cytometry

4.5.1. Lymphocyte Phenotyping

Peripheral blood lymphocyte analysis using the CD markers for T-cells ($CD2^+$), T-helper cells ($CD4^+$) and T-cytotoxic suppressor cells ($CD8^+$) was performed by a flow cytometer (Coulter Epics XL 4C, Beckman Coulter Company, Brea, CA, USA) according to the method described previously by Dudek et al. [18].

4.5.2. Phagocytic Activity and Oxygen Metabolism of Leukocytes

Phagocytic activity and oxygen metabolism of peripheral blood leukocytes were evaluated according to the manufacturer's instructions of two separated commercial kits: Phagotest™ for leukocyte phagocytic activity and Phagoburst™ for oxygen metabolism analysis, both manufactured by Glycotope Biotechnology GmbH (Heidelberg, Germany) and analyzed using Epics XL flow cytometer (Beckman Coulter, Miami, FL, USA). The granulocyte and monocyte phagocytic activity was expressed as the percentage of cells that engulfed bacteria as well as mean fluorescence intensity (MFI) of the cells for estimating of phagocytosed bacteria amount. The oxygen metabolism of peripheral blood leukocytes was determined as the percentage of cells activated by *E. coli* as well as MFI for the measurement of phagocytic activity of leukocytes.

4.6. Immunohistochemistry

The collected lung samples were examined using an immunohistochemical staining for the detection of local immune response markers such as CD3 (T-cells), CD79 (B-cells), MHC class II and S100. Previously prepared sections were deparaffinized in xylene, rehydrated in descending ethanol concentrations, then incubated in 3% H_2O_2 diluted in methanol for 10 min and submitted to heat-induced epitope retrieval in citrate buffer (pH 6.0) using a pressure cooker for 20 min. Depending on the marker the slides were then incubated for one hour with primary antibodies as follows: rabbit anti-CD3 monoclonal antibody (A045201, DAKO, Glostrup, Denmark) at dilution 1:100 for CD3 detection; mouse monoclonal anti-CD79a antibody [HM57] (ab62650, Abcam, Cambridge, UK) at dilution 1:400 for CD79a detection; mouse anti-HLA-DR Antigen, Alpha-Chain, Clone TAL.1B5 (M074601-2, DAKO, Glostrup, Denmark) at dilution 1:40 for MHC class II detection and FLEX Polyclonal

Rb anti-S100, RTU (GA50461-2, DAKO) at dilution 1:1 for S100 detection. The antibody detection was performed using the Dako REAL EnVision Detection System, Peroxidase/DAB, Rabbit/Mouse (K5007, DAKO, Glostrup, Denmark), involving an incubation with a peroxidase-conjugated polymer as a secondary antibody (for 30 min) and DAB^{+} Chromogen applied for a visualization of the reaction. Sections were counterstained with Mayer's hematoxylin, dehydrated and mounted. Sections incubated with PBS instead of the primary antibody were used to confirm the specificity of the staining. The tissues were analyzed under a light microscope (Axiolab, Zeiss, Oberkochen, Germany) for the presence of brown staining indicating positive labeling of *M. bovis*, CD3, CD79a, MHC class II and S100. To determine the difference between the number of T- and B-lymphocytes infiltrating the tissue in the examined sections of experimental group and to compare number of the two cell–type populations between the experimental and control groups, the CD3- and CD79a-positive cells were counted in 20 high power fields (400x) comprising the cell infiltrations and/or BALT in each slide.

4.7. Statistical Analysis

The results are presented as arithmetic means or mean percentage ± standard deviation. The differences between the mean values recorded in the E and C groups at the same time point were analyzed using *t*-test with a statistically significant level of $p < 0.05$. The same test and the *p*-value were applied to determine the difference between the mean values of summarized cell counts for the CD3 and CD79a markers analyzed with IHC in the experimental and control groups.

Supplementary Materials: The following are available online at http://www.mdpi.com/2076-0817/9/5/407/s1, Figure S1. Numerical values for hematology; Figure S2. Numerical values for lymphocyte phenotyping; Figure S3. Numerical values for phagocytic activity of granulocytes; Figure S4. Numerical values for phagocytic activity of monocytes; Figure S5. Numerical values for oxygen metabolism of leukocytes.

Author Contributions: Conceptualization, K.D. and D.B.; methodology, K.D., A.K., U.L., M.R.; formal analysis, K.D., A.K., U.L.; investigation, K.D., A.K., U.L., D.B. and technical staff; writing—original draft preparation, K.D. and partially A.K.; writing—review and editing, D.B. and U.L.; supervision, D.B., M.R., K.K., S.W.; project administration, K.D.; funding acquisition, K.D., D.B., K.K., M.R. All authors have read and agreed to the published version of the manuscript.

Funding: The immunohistochemical analyses for CD3, CD79a, MHCII and S100 detection in the lung tissues were performed within the project entitled 'Improving methods for identifying *Mycoplasma bovis* infections in cattle and assessing the development of the immune response with its participation in enzootic calf bronchopneumonia' funded by Krajowy Naukowy Osrodek Wiodacy - KNOW (Leading National Research Center) Scientific Consortium "Healthy Animal—Safe Food", decision of Ministry of Science and Higher Education No. 05-1/KNOW2/2015.

Conflicts of Interest: The authors declare no conflict of interest.

References

1. Adegboye, D.S.; Halbur, P.G.; Nutsch, R.G.; Kadlec, R.G.; Rosenbusch, R.F. *Mycoplasma bovis*-associated pneumonia and arthritis complicated with pyogranulomatous tenosynovitis in calves. *J. Am. Vet. Med. Assoc.* **1996**, *209*, 647–649. [PubMed]
2. Caswell, J.L.; Archambault, M. *Mycoplasma bovis* pneumonia in cattle. *Anim. Health Res. Rev.* **2009**, *8*, 161–186. [CrossRef] [PubMed]
3. Nicholas, R.A.; Ayling, R.D. *Mycoplasma bovis*: Disease, diagnosis, and control. *Res. Vet. Sci.* **2003**, *74*, 105–112. [CrossRef]
4. Srikumaran, S.; Kelling, C.L.; Ambagala, A. Immune evasion by pathogens of bovine respiratory disease complex. *Anim. Health Res. Rev.* **2008**, *8*, 215–229. [CrossRef] [PubMed]
5. Jungi, T.W.; Krampe, M.; Sileghem, M.; Griot, C.; Nicolet, J. Differential and strain-specific triggering of bovine alveolar macrophage effector functions by mycoplasmas. *Microb. Pathog.* **1996**, *21*, 487–498. [CrossRef] [PubMed]
6. Jimbo, S.; Suleman, M.; Maina, T.; Prysliak, T.; Mulongo, M.; Perez-Casal, J. Effect of *Mycoplasma bovis* on bovine neutrophils. *Vet. Immunol. Immunopathol.* **2017**, *188*, 27–33. [CrossRef] [PubMed]

7. Thomas, C.B.; Van Ess, P.; Wolfgram, L.J.; Riebe, J.; Sharp, P.; Schultz, R.D. Adherence to bovine neutrophils and suppression of neutrophil chemiluminescence by *Mycoplasma bovis*. *Vet. Immunol. Immunopathol.* **1991**, *27*, 365–381. [CrossRef]
8. Thomas, C.B.; Mettler, J.; Sharp, P.; Jensen-Kostenbader, J.; Schultz, R.D. *Mycoplasma bovis* suppression of bovine lymphocyte response to phytohemagglutinin. *Vet. Immunol. Immunopathol.* **1990**, *26*, 143–155. [CrossRef]
9. Vanden Bush, T.J.; Rosenbusch, R.F. Characterization of a lympho-inhibitory peptide produced by *Mycoplasma bovis*. *Biochem. Biophys. Res. Commun.* **2004**, *315*, 336–341. [CrossRef] [PubMed]
10. Hermeyer, K.; Buchenau, I.; Thomasmeyer, A.; Baum, B.; Spergser, J.; Rosengarten, R.; Hewicker-Trautwein, M. Chronic pneumonia in calves after experimental infection with *Mycoplasma bovis* strain 1067: Characterization of lung pathology, persistence of variable surface protein antigens and local immune response. *Acta Vet. Scand.* **2012**, *54*, 9–11. [CrossRef] [PubMed]
11. Hermeyer, K.; Peters, M.; Brügmann, M.; Jacobsen, B.; Hewicker-Trautwein, M. Demonstration of *Mycoplasma bovis* by immunohistochemistry and in situ hybridization in an aborted bovine fetus and neonatal calf. *J. Vet. Diagn. Investig.* **2012**, *24*, 364–369. [CrossRef] [PubMed]
12. Dudek, K.; Bednarek, D.; Ayling, R.D.; Kycko, A.; Reichert, M. Preliminary study on the effects of enrofloxacin, flunixin meglumine and pegbovigrastim on *Mycoplasma bovis* pneumonia. *BMC Vet. Res.* **2019**, *15*, 371–384. [CrossRef] [PubMed]
13. Khodakaram-Tafti, A.; López, A. Immunohistopathological findings in the lungs of calves naturally infected with *Mycoplasma bovis*. *J. Vet. Med. A Physiol. Pathol. Clin. Med.* **2004**, *51*, 10–14. [CrossRef] [PubMed]
14. Kleinschmidt, S.; Spergser, J.; Rosengarten, R.; Hewicker-Trautwein, M. Long-term survival of *Mycoplasma bovis* in necrotic lesions and in phagocytic cells as demonstrated by transmission and immunogold electron microscopy in lung tissue from experimentally infected calves. *Vet. Microbiol.* **2013**, *162*, 949–953. [CrossRef] [PubMed]
15. Gondaira, S.; Higuchi, H.; Nishi, K.; Iwano, H.; Nagahata, H. *Mycoplasma bovis* escapes bovine neutrophil extracellular traps. *Vet. Microbiol.* **2017**, *199*, 68–73. [CrossRef] [PubMed]
16. Howard, C.J.; Taylor, G.; Collins, J.; Gourlay, R.N. Interaction of *Mycoplasma dispar* and *Mycoplasma agalactiae* subsp. *bovis* with bovine alveolar macrophages and bovine lacteal polymorphonuclear leukocytes. *Infect. Immun.* **1976**, *14*, 11–17. [CrossRef] [PubMed]
17. Wiggins, M.C.; Woolums, A.R.; Hurley, D.J.; Sanchez, S.; Ensley, D.T.; Donovan, D. The effect of various *Mycoplasma bovis* isolates on bovine leukocyte responses. *Comp. Immunol. Microbiol. Infect. Dis.* **2011**, *34*, 49–54. [CrossRef] [PubMed]
18. Dudek, K.; Bednarek, D.; Szacawa, E.; Rosales, R.S.; Ayling, R.D. Flow cytometry follow-up analysis of peripheral blood leukocyte subpopulations in calves experimentally infected with field isolates of *Mycoplasma bovis*. *Acta Vet. Hung.* **2015**, *63*, 167–178. [CrossRef] [PubMed]

pathogens

MDPI

Article

Field Experience of Antibody Testing against *Mycoplasma bovis* in Adult Cows in Commercial Danish Dairy Cattle Herds

Mette Bisgaard Petersen [1,*], Lars Pedersen [2], Lone Møller Pedersen [3] and Liza Rosenbaum Nielsen [4]

1 Department of Veterinary Clinical Sciences, University of Copenhagen, Agrovej 5A, 2630 Taastrup, Denmark
2 SEGES, 8200 Aarhus, Denmark; larp@seges.dk
3 Eurofins Milk Testing Denmark, 6600 Vejen, Denmark; lonemollerpedersen@eurofins.dk
4 Department of Animal and Veterinary Sciences, University of Copenhagen, Grønnegårdsvej 8, 1870 Frederiksberg, Denmark; liza@sund.ku.dk
* Correspondence: mbp@sund.ku.dk

Received: 30 June 2020; Accepted: 3 August 2020; Published: 6 August 2020

Abstract: *Mycoplasma bovis* in cattle is difficult to diagnose. Recently, the ID screen® mycoplasma bovis indirect ELISA (ID screen) was commercially released by IDVet. The objectives of this study were to: (1) gain and share experience of using the ID screen in adult dairy cows under field conditions; (2) determine the correlation between antibody levels in milk and serum and (3) compare the ID screen results with those of the Bio K 302 (BioX 302) ELISA from BioX Diagnostics. Paired serum and milk samples were collected from 270 cows from 12 Danish dairy herds with three categories of *M. bovis* disease history. The ID screen tested nearly all cows positive in all, but the three non-infected herds, while the BioX 302 tested very few cows positive. The ID screen is therefore a much more sensitive test than the BioX 302. However, cows in five exposed herds without signs of ongoing infection and two herds with no history of *M. bovis* infection also tested ID screen positive. Therefore, the performance and interpretation of the test must be investigated under field conditions in best practice test evaluation setups. A concordance correlation coefficient of 0.66 (95% CI: 0.59–0.72) between the ID screen serum and milk results indicates that milk samples can replace serum samples for the ID screen diagnosis of *M. bovis* in adult cows.

Keywords: *Mycoplasma bovis*; diagnosis; control; immune response; ELISA

1. Introduction

Mycoplasma bovis (*M. bovis*) is an emerging bacterium associated with disease in cattle of all ages in many countries around the world [1]. In dairy cows, the usual presentation is mastitis, pneumonia and/or arthritis, while calves typically suffer from pneumonia, otitis media and/or arthritis [2,3]. Diagnosing *M. bovis* is challenging at both animal and herd level. *M. bovis*-associated disease can be diagnosed by using bacterial culture or PCR on body fluids or organ specimens and antibody measurements in serum or milk [3]. However, the fact that *M. bovis* bacteria lead to so many different disease manifestations and varying test responses in different age groups, and the fact that there is not one single diagnostic material that can test for and differentiate between all these disease manifestations makes it difficult to diagnose *M. bovis*-associated disease [4].

Antibody tests are inexpensive and for some purposes, it is an advantage that they can also detect previous (recent) infection. The first and previously only commercially available test for antibodies directed against *M. bovis* was produced by BioX Diagnostics in Belgium. The Bio K 302 ELISA kit (BioX 302) has been reported to have low sensitivity ranging from 0.37–0.50 and specificity ranging from 0.90–0.96 in experimental studies [5–7] and very short-lasting antibody detection in individual cows [8] and calves [9]. Petersen et al. [8] found that the mean antibody level in cows with clinical indication of *M. bovis* was only above the recommended cutoff (37 ODC%) for approximately 60 days after the disease outbreak, which implies that frequent testing would be necessary to detect disease among cows if the BioX 302 were to be used to assess the *M. bovis* status of dairy cows or herds. One explanation could be the large antigenic variation of *M. bovis* and the alterations of membrane surface lipoproteins over time [10]. Studies have compared the BioX 302 to an in-house *M. bovis* ELISA based on a different antigen. The agreement between the results from the two tests was low, and the antibodies detected by the in-house ELISA persisted in serum from cows 1.5 years after the disease outbreak regardless of the current *M. bovis* clinical status [9,11]. Results from one ELISA test can therefore not be extrapolated to other *M. bovis*-detecting ELISAs. The differences in test performance may be influenced by the different antigens used in each ELISA, how immunogenic they are, how long the immune system reacts to the particular protein and how similar the gene of that particular protein is in different *M. bovis* strains.

The ID screen® mycoplasma bovis indirect (ID screen) from IDvet (Grabels, France) is a reasonably new commercially available antibody test. According to the manufacturer, the diagnostic sensitivity and specificity are 95.7% and 100%, respectively [12]. The test has only been evaluated in calves [12], but the age of the animals is very likely to influence the test performance when used under field conditions [13,14]. Therefore, current knowledge about the ID screen test performance may not be valid for adult cows and may vary depending on whether the test material is serum or milk.

Applying the BioX 302 to herd-level testing using bulk tank milk has been evaluated and found useful in estimating the prevalence at a national level when the cutoff was raised to 55 ODC% [15]. However, the challenge is that bulk tank milk primarily reflects *M. bovis* udder infections in the herd [8]. In fact, one study found that the hospital herd was the most indicative group to use for the detection of herd-level *M. bovis* infection based on bulk tank milk tested using the BioX 302 [16]. Danish cattle farmers have experienced many *M. bovis* disease outbreaks characterized by arthritis rather than mastitis as the primary clinical sign [8], and bulk tank milk samples would most likely fail to detect these outbreaks. Use of the BioX 302 on milk samples is non-optimal due to the need for frequent testing to ensure infected herds are detected (e.g., for classification of herds in relation to trade, shows, etc.), and because not all disease manifestations can be detected when measuring antibodies in milk [4,16]. As the ID screen is more sensitive than BioX 302, antibody measurements in milk may be more reliable, potentially making it feasible to use antibody testing of individual and bulk tank milk samples for surveillance or outbreak diagnostics, providing the specificity is sufficiently high. The potential use of ELISA on milk samples to classify or monitor dairy herds for *M. bovis* infection will be of interest in a setting like the Danish dairy industry, since the sampling can be automated via the mandatory milk quality control scheme and bulk tank milk surveillance for other cattle diseases.

The objectives of this study were therefore to: (1) gain and share experience of using the new commercial ELISA ID screen for the detection of antibodies against *M. bovis* in adult dairy cows under field conditions; (2) determine the correlation between the measured antibody levels in milk and serum and (3) compare the ID screen results with the results of the frequently used and commercially available BioX 302 ELISA.

2. Results

Paired serum and milk samples were collected from a total of 270 cows from 12 Danish dairy herds. All nasal swabs and milk samples from lactating cows in the Robust Calves herds (RC-herds) tested negative for the presence of *M. bovis* by PCR. See Table 1 and the Section 4 for a description of the different herds included in the study.

The serum and milk ID screen sample-to-positive percentage (S/P%) was plotted with jittered dots for each of the 12 herds (Figures 1 and 2). All cows had a S/P% below the recommended cutoff in both serum and milk in three herds (herds 1–3). In all other herds, all or nearly all cows had a S/P% above the recommended cutoff.

The serum and milk BioX 302 sample-coefficient (ODC%) was plotted with jittered dots for each of the 12 herds (Figures 3 and 4). All, but 16 cows from seven different herds had serum ODC% values below the recommended cutoff in serum, while all, but 17 cows from nine different herds had milk ODC% values below the recommended cutoff.

Correlation between Serum and Milk S/P%

The concordance correlation coefficient between serum and milk S/P% across the full dataset of paired serum and milk samples was 0.66 (95% CI: 0.59–0.72). The correlation between serum and milk samples within each herd is shown in Figure 5. Correlations are not shown for the BioX 302 due to the low number of positive samples.

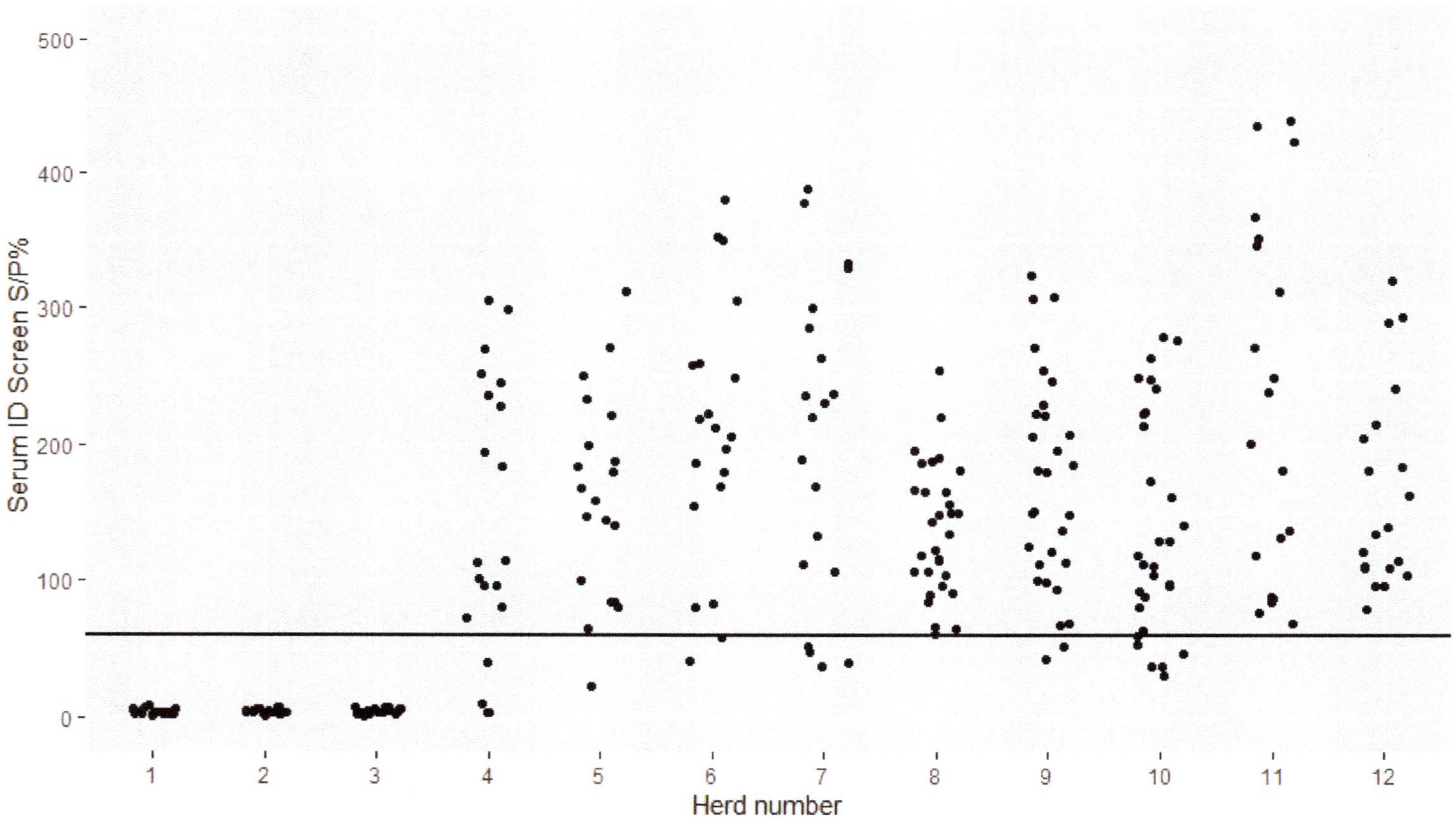

Figure 1. Serum antibody levels against *Mycoplasma bovis* in cows from 12 Danish dairy herds tested with the ID screen® mycoplasma bovis indirect ELISA kit from IDvet. Herds 1–6 and 11–12 had 20 cows tested and herds 8–10 had 30 cows tested. The horizontal black line indicates the manufacturer-recommended cutoff value (sample-to-positive percentage (S/P%) of 60) for serum.

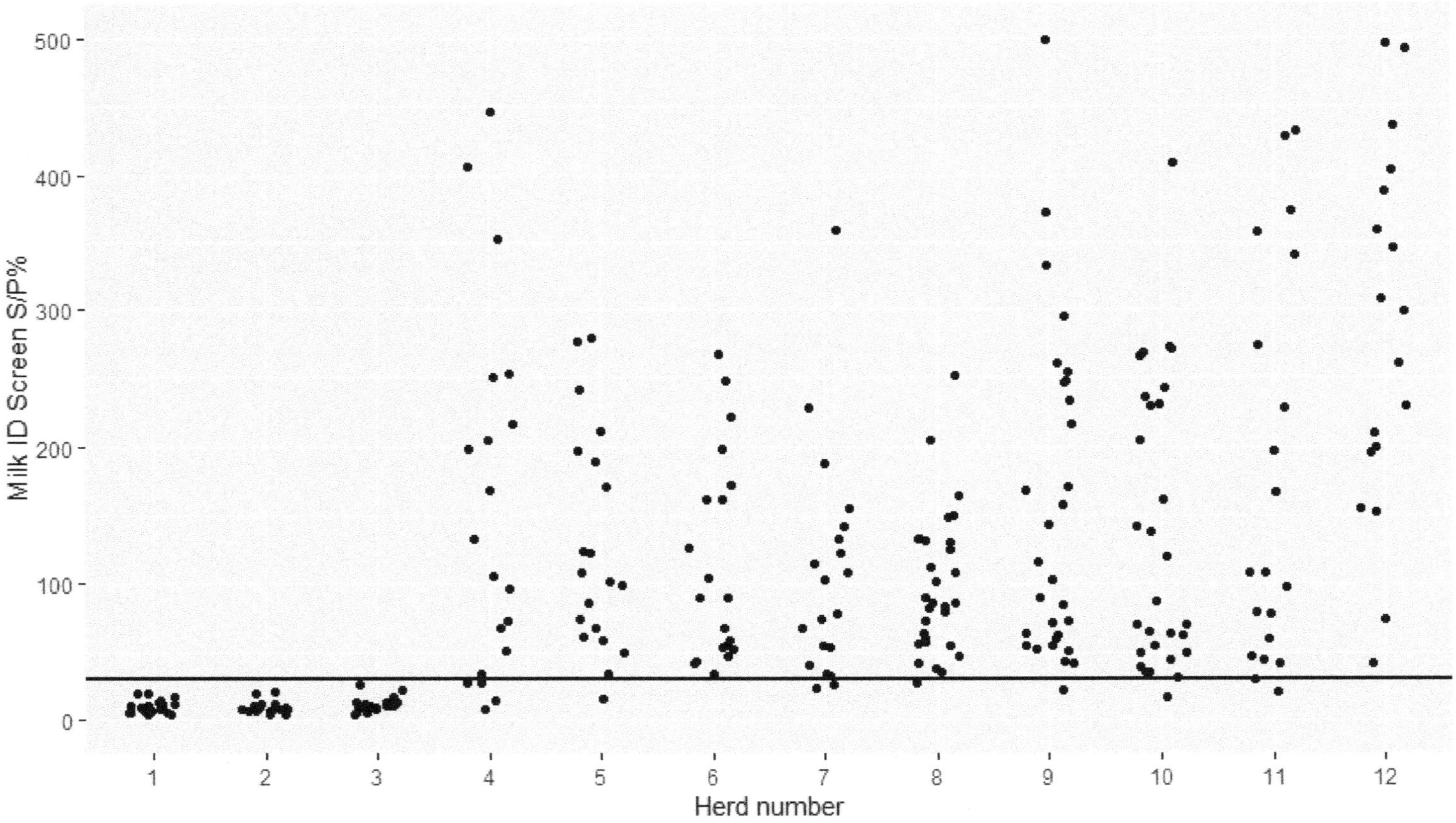

Figure 2. Milk antibody levels against *Mycoplasma bovis* in cows from 12 Danish dairy herds tested with the ID screen® mycoplasma bovis indirect ELISA kit from IDvet. Herds 1–6 and 11–12 had 20 cows tested and Herds 8–10 had 30 cows tested. The horizontal black line indicates the manufacturer-recommended cutoff value (sample-to-positive percentage (S/P%) of 30) for the overnight protocol for milk.

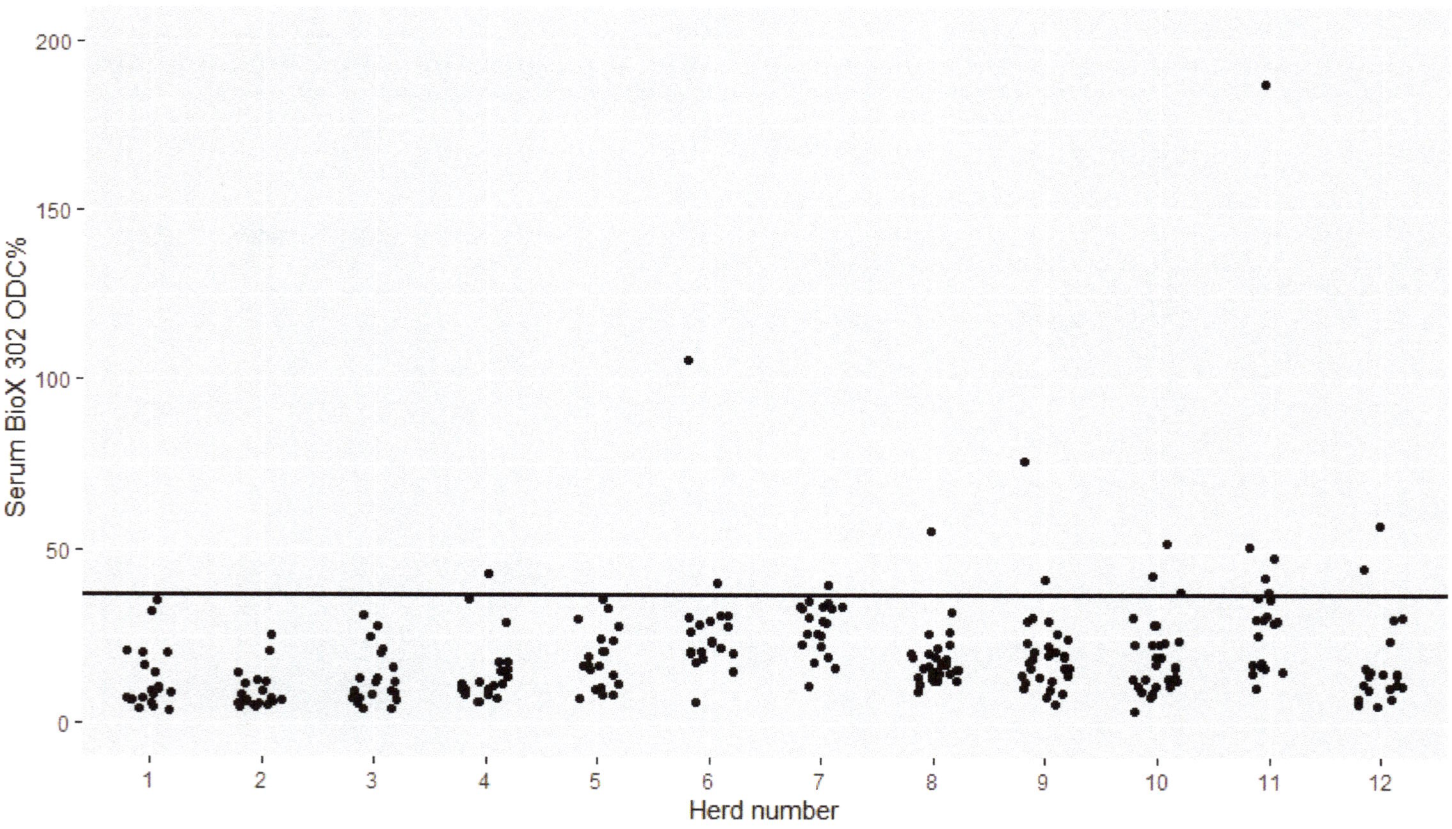

Figure 3. Serum antibody levels against *Mycoplasma bovis* in cows from 12 Danish dairy herds tested with the Bio K 302 ELISA kit from BioX. Herds 1–6 and 11–12 had 20 cows tested and Herds 8–10 had 30 cows tested. The horizontal black line indicates the manufacturer-recommended cutoff value (sample-coefficient (ODC%) of 37).

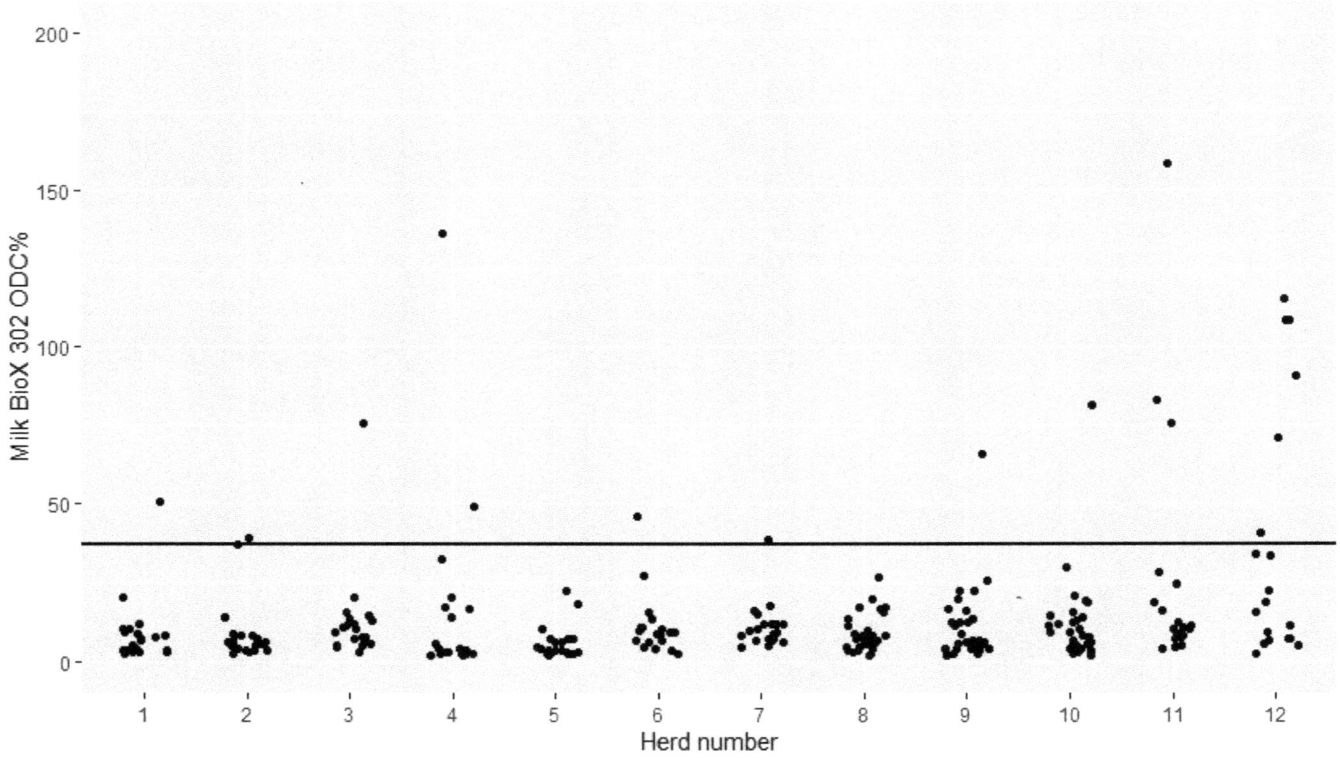

Figure 4. Milk antibody levels against *Mycoplasma bovis* in cows from 12 Danish dairy herds tested with the Bio K 302 ELISA kit from BioX. Herds 1–6 and 11–12 had 20 cows tested and Herds 8–10 had 30 cows tested. The horizontal black line indicates the manufacturer-recommended cutoff value (sample-coefficient (ODC%) of 37).

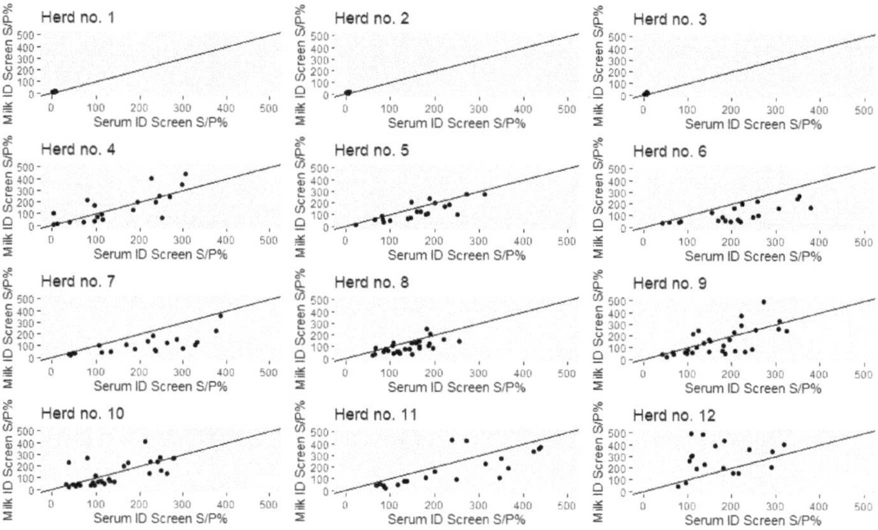

Figure 5. Correlations between paired serum and milk sample-to-positive percentage (S/P%) against *Mycoplasma bovis* using the ID screen® mycoplasma bovis indirect ELISA kit, stratified across 12 Danish dairy herds. The diagonal line indicates perfect agreement between serum and milk values.

3. Discussion

In the present study, we tested milk and serum samples from cows in Danish dairy herds for which we had prior knowledge of the *M. bovis* infection status, in order to gain and share experience of using the ID screen for detecting antibodies against *M. bovis* in adult dairy cows under field conditions and to compare the results with the results of BioX 302. We also determined the correlation between the measured antibody levels in milk and serum for the ID screen across the full dataset of 12 dairy herds and inspected visualizations of the different correlation patterns for the individual herds.

3.1. Field Performance of the ID Screen and BioX 302

Overall, many cows and most of the herds tested positive in both serum and milk when the ID screen was used (Figures 1 and 2). In only three of the 12 herds (Herds 1–3), all samples were negative in both serum and milk. These herds were all previously classified as not infected with *M. bovis*, indicating good concordance between the classification and the test results for these three herds. However, herds 4 and 5 were also classified as not infected, but most both serum and milk samples were positive. This is interesting and there could be several reasons for this, as discussed below.

With regard to the five herds classified as infected with *M. bovis* within the last 5 years (Herds 6–10), nearly all cows tested positive using the ID screen, despite the fact that none of the farmers thought that they had ongoing disease problems related to *M. bovis* at sampling. Four of the herds had an *M. bovis* disease outbreak 4–5 years prior to sampling. Most sampled cows in the three Outbreak-herds had not been born at the time of the disease outbreak. The persistence of antibodies in these herds therefore suggests that the cows were still exposed to *M. bovis*, despite not showing clinical signs around the time of sampling in this study. The two RC-herds classified as infected within the last 5 years both had calves that tested positive for antibodies in both the ID screen and BioX 302, as well as positive PCR samples. In these herds, it is more apparent that the animals were probably exposed to *M. bovis* around the time of sampling. If milk samples and nasal swabs for PCR-testing had been collected from the Outbreak-herds, it cannot be ruled out that some of them would have been positive as well, indicating a recent exposure to *M. bovis* despite there being no sign of disease.

The two herds classified as infected at the time of sampling both had all, but one sample above the cutoff and some of the highest S/P% seen in this study. This makes good sense in terms of the classification, and there was good concordance between the classification and test results in these herds. There was ongoing *M. bovis* infection at least among the calves, where the positive PCR samples were collected. However, none of the PCR tests from nasal swabs or milk samples collected from cows were positive. These were samples from healthy cows, and it cannot be ruled out that if the same samples had been collected from diseased cows, an indication of *M. bovis* infection may have been observed among the cows [4,16].

None of the study herds had ongoing clinical signs of an *M. bovis* disease outbreak. However, the herds still tested positive using the ID screen. All sampled cows were considered to be healthy by the farmer, were housed in the main milking herd and delivered milk to the bulk tank on the day of sampling. Based on this, it is not possible to use the ID screen to differentiate between healthy and diseased cows, but it is likely that the ID screen tests for exposure to *M. bovis*. Cattle can be subclinically infected with *M. bovis* [3], and if the ID screen tests positive in subclinically infected animals, it is potentially a very useful test to use in relation to prevent the spread of infection. However, further studies are needed as this study did not determine the *M. bovis* status of the individual cow, but the herd as a whole.

The ID screen is a sensitive test, as all or nearly all cows in each herd tested either positive or negative. This makes the test good for herd-level control and surveillance purposes, as a small sample of cows would give a good indication of the exposure status of the age group as a whole. However, there may be issues with the diagnostic (field-use) specificity of ID screen, as many of the cows in two out of the five herds classified as not infected within the previous 5 years prior to sampling did test positive. A possible explanation could be that the tested cows in the herds classified as non-infected had been subclinically infected [3] and had therefore never shown any clinical signs. The historical serologic herd classification for this study was based on the BioX 302, which primarily detects clinically ill animals [8,16]. The specificity under field conditions must therefore be investigated further, preferably in field studies based on best practice diagnostic test evaluation [17].

The BioX 302 showed a rather different test pattern. In general, most of the serum and milk samples tested negative. However, there were a small number of positive serum and milk samples in some herds (Figures 3 and 4). The BioX 302 has been shown to have a poor sensitivity [5] and to primarily detect clinically ill animals [8,16]. Taking these findings into account, it is not surprising that the cows in this study generally tested negative when using the BioX 302, as only two herds were classified as having an ongoing *M. bovis* infection. The few positive test results were found in all three herd classifications (not infected, infected within the last 5 years and infected at sampling), and in particular, few positive results were found in milk samples from the non-infected herds (Figures 3 and 4). Herd 4 was classified as not infected but had one positive serum sample and two positive milk samples, one of which was very high in ODC% (140). This could suggest subclinical mastitis in these cows, although they were not positive in PCR on milk. Herds 11 and 12 were classified as having an ongoing *M. bovis* infection, and both of these herds tested positive in a low number of serum and milk samples tested using BioX 302, and this was most pronounced in milk samples. Again, this could suggest subclinical mastitis cases in these herds. Based on the PCR samples from calves (Table 1), it seems that at least this age group was infected with *M. bovis* in herds 11 and 12. It would have been interesting to see the results of the BioX 302 on serum samples from calves—and whether this method would have detected the infection among calves. However, we have previously shown that the BioX 302 did not detect antibodies in calves exposed to *M. bovis* before 3 months of age [9], and all of the samples from the RC-project (Robust Calves project) are from calves under 3 months of age. Previous results have shown that the disease status among calves is not reflected in the bulk tank milk [18], and the findings of this study support that *M. bovis* infection in young stock cannot be measured using the BioX 302 in serum or milk samples from the cows either.

In comparison, there are very large differences in the test patterns between ID screen and BioX 302. Nearly all cows in all, but three non-infected herds were found to be positive when using the ID screen, while in contrast, very few cows tested positive using the BioX 302. As discussed above, the ID screen is a much more sensitive test than the BioX 302 and may be able to detect subclinically infected animals [3], as opposed to the BioX 302, which primarily detects diseased animals [8]. However, nearly all cows tested positive in herds without an ongoing infection, as well as in herds with no history of *M. bovis* infection. This leads to the hypothesis that the ID screen will measure exposure to *M. bovis* rather than colonization and dissemination of the organism in the infected animal. Whatever the reason for the very different test patterns, the interpretation and recommendations for the use of ID screen must be different from that of the BioX 302.

3.2. Correlation between Serum and Milk Samples

The concordance correlation coefficient between serum and milk S/P% was 0.66 (95% CI: 0.59–0.72). In general, the serum values were higher than the milk values, except in herd 12 (Figure 5). This could be explained by different clinical manifestations, e.g., clinical or subclinical mastitis cases could induce mostly high milk S/P% and systemic disease could induce mostly high serum S/P%, as previously shown when using the BioX 302 test [8]. This may also be the case for the ID screen, but to a lesser degree since the cows still test positive in both serum and milk.

The clinical signs present in the Outbreak-herds (herds 8–10) during the *M. bovis* disease outbreak are known as they were part of another *M. bovis* project. Herd 8 had many cows with clinical signs of arthritis and no *M. bovis* PCR-positive milk samples, while herds 9 and 10 experienced a combination of arthritis and mastitis among the cows. Herd 8 had clearly higher S/P% in serum than milk, while herds 9 and 10 had some very high milk values (Figure 5). Even though 4–5 years had passed since the *M. bovis* disease outbreak, the initial clinical expression may still be evident in the ID screen results. If this is the case, it is likely that herd 12 had subclinical mastitis cases.

The observed correlation between ID screen serum and milk values suggests that milk samples may be a promising replacement for serum samples. Strong responses observed in individual cows are also promising signs for the potential use of ID screen on bulk tank milk samples for herd-level diagnosis. This would be advantageous for surveillance and control purposes and for sampling many cows, since milk samples are easier and cheaper to collect than blood samples.

3.3. Uncertainty in Herd Classification

Herd classification is, among other things, based on previous BioX 302 tests and PCR on individual and bulk tank milk samples. The bulk tank milk samples were primarily collected as yearly surveillance tests and are therefore not sampled often enough to ensure the detection of new and mild infections– in the case of an *M. bovis* infection, the detectable response in bulk tank milk can be very short-lived for both BioX 302 and PCR [4,16]. It is possible that some of the herds could have had a previous *M. bovis* infection that was not detected in bulk tank milk by either BioX 302 or PCR, especially if the clinical signs were not severe and the farmer had not collected additional samples.

Herd 2 was classified as not infected despite one positive PCR sample and two positive BioX 302 serum samples, all from calves. The positive PCR test was one out of 209 tested samples. Taking into account that the PCR test is not 100% specific [19], this was judged to be a false positive result. Overall, based on the uncertainties in the diagnostic tests and no other indications of previous or current *M. bovis* infection, we have chosen to classify this herd as not infected.

The farmer from Herd 5 stated that the herd had experienced an *M. bovis* disease outbreak in 2012. It is possible that the ID screen would still be able to detect this exposure, even though seven years had passed since the disease outbreak. However, it is noteworthy that the calves did not test positive in the ID screen, despite calves often being the reservoir of the infection [3]. As discussed above, the BioX 302 is not a sensitive test in young calves, but an in-house ELISA with another antigen (MilA) has been evaluated with good sensitivity in young calves [9], indicating that another ELISA could perform better than the BioX 302 in calves. Based on the ID screen and PCR tests of calves, it seems likely that the young calves were not infected with *M. bovis*, and transmission must therefore occur among older calves in Herd 5. This implies that the milk management and separation of cows from young calves must be adequate in hindering transmission to the young calves. In this herd, the calves were born in a common calving pen and left with the cow for at least 12 h. The calves were then moved to single pens outside, very well separated from the cows. This management may have been sufficient to stop the young calves being exposed, even though there was infection among the cows. In Herd 4, none of the available tests were positive and the farmer stated that the herd had not had an *M. bovis* disease outbreak. This also highlights the difficulties in assessing infection with *M. bovis*. If the positive results of the ID screen are truly a sign of ongoing *M. bovis* infection or exposure within that herd, then it is a very difficult organism to detect. With nearly all cows testing positive in both serum and milk, we find it unlikely that these would be false positive samples. It could be that the ID screen cross-reacts with antibodies against other mycoplasma species. The importance of testing for cross-reactivity with other *Mycoplasma* spp., especially *M. agalactiae*, has been emphasized for other *M. bovis* ELISAs [20], however no such information can be found in the documentation for the ID screen [12,21].

4. Materials and Methods

4.1. Study Herds

Herds were selected for participation based on the availability of prior information about the *M. bovis* status. Information from dairy herds participating in two other research projects as well as knowledge from test results from previously collected samples made it possible to include herds known to have had an *M. bovis* outbreak and herds that had not had an outbreak (Table 1). Nine herds were included due to their participation in a large Danish calf-health research project ('Robust calves project' running from 2018–2021 in which nasal swabs, tracheal washes and blood samples were collected from randomly selected calves across three age groups). These herds are referred to as the RC-herds. The remaining three herds were included because they were known to have had an *M. bovis* disease outbreak with test-positive samples while participating in an *M. bovis* research project 3–4 years prior to the initiation of the present study [8]. These three herds are referred to as the Outbreak-herds.

There was variation among herds in how difficult it was to determine the present and previous *M. bovis* status and additional samples and diagnostic test history were therefore also included from on-farm animal health monitoring activities in order to facilitate the grouping of herds. Details are shown in Table 1.

Previous individual and bulk tank milk *M. bovis* PCR and ELISA results were confirmed from the Danish Cattle Database, which is a national cattle register for all Danish cattle herds. Both national surveillance and diagnostic tests voluntarily conducted on the request of the local veterinarian and farmers are registered here, and we included the available data from 2012–2019. PCR-tested milk samples from which results were available in the Danish Cattle Database were analyzed using the Pathoproof Major-3 or Complete-16 assays (Thermo Scientific, Waltham, MA) or Mastit 4 (DNA Diagnostic, Risskov, Denmark); the ELISA test used was the BioX 302.

Blood samples were collected from many calves in the RC-herds on several occasions during autumn and winter 2019 and 2020 as part of another project. To better characterize potential *M. bovis* infection in these herds, approximately 30 blood samples from seven of these herds were analyzed with the ID screen and BioX 302. During the RC-project, nasal swabs and tracheal washes were also collected from between 129 and 431 calves in each RC-herd (see Table 1 for details), and they were all tested for the presence of *M. bovis* with the Fluidigm PCR test (see Laboratory Analysis for details). No additional diagnostic tests were performed in the three Outbreak-herds.

On the basis of all the information gathered—and considering the fact that the sensitivity and specificity of the BioX 302 ELISA and the Fluidigm PCR tests are not perfect [5,6,19]—all herds were classified as either:

- Not infected—meaning that none (or very few, likely false positives) of the available test results were positive for *M. bovis* and the farmer stated that they had never had clinical signs of *M. bovis*-associated disease or that the clinical signs occurred more than 5 years prior to sampling;
- Infected within the last 5 years—meaning that there were multiple positive diagnostic test results in previously or recently collected samples and/or reporting of clinical signs of *M. bovis* within the last 5 years prior to sampling;
- Infected at sampling—meaning that diagnostic tests indicated an ongoing infection with *M. bovis* among one or more age groups at the time of sampling for the present study.

4.2. Sample Collection

Paired serum and milk samples were collected from cows from the 12 dairy herds during the first quarter of 2019. For all nine RC-herds, paired blood and milk samples were collected from 20 lactating dairy cows, and a nasal swab was collected from the same cows for the detection of *M. bovis*. We aimed to collect samples from primiparous cows, but it was not practically feasible in all herds (Herds 1, 2 and 3), so older cows were also included in the sample collection. The blood samples were collected from the coccygeal vein in plain serum tubes. Prior to milk sampling, the teats were cleaned with ethanol on a tissue, the first milk was discarded and a composite milk sample consisting of milk from all udder quarters was collected from each cow in a bronopol-coated tube to preserve the milk sample. The nasal swabs were taken with a long sterile cotton swab, rubbed gently against the mucosa in one naris until saturated and placed in phosphate-buffered saline until analysis.

All procedures involving animals in this study were conducted in accordance with guidelines from the Danish Ministry of Justice with respect to animal experimentation and care of animals under study (The Danish Ministry of Justice, 2014, LBK no. 474). The Danish Animal Experiments Inspectorate under the Danish Veterinary and Food Administration was consulted for guidance on required permissions and approved the project activities in writing without requiring further formal application or approval processes. Following sampling of the animals, all herd owners were interviewed about their perception and experience with *M. bovis*-associated disease at their farm (summarized in Table 1).

Paired blood and milk samples were collected from 30 cows from the Outbreak-herds. No further tests were done in these herds as they were all known to have had a confirmed outbreak of *M. bovis*-associated disease in 2015–2016.

The number of cows included in each herd was optimized according to the available budget.

The serum and milk samples were analyzed for antibodies against *M. bovis* using the ID screen and the BioX 302. Following antibody analysis, the milk samples were frozen and stored for approximately 6 months and then tested for the presence of *M. bovis* bacterial DNA using the commercial PCR Pathoproof Major-3 assay. The nasal swabs were analyzed for the presence of *M. bovis* using the Fluidigm PCR system.

4.3. Laboratory Analysis

For the ID screen, a S/P% $\geq$ 60 for the serum sample was considered positive and for the milk samples the overnight incubation protocol was used in order to optimize the sensitivity and the samples were considered positive if S/P% $\geq$ 30 [12]. For the BIO K 302, an ODC% $\geq$ 37 was considered positive [22]. The Pathoproof Major-3 assay (Thermo Scientific, Waltham, MA, USA) and the Mastit 4 PCR assay (DNA diagnostic, Risskov, Denmark) were considered positive if the cycle threshold (Ct) value < 37. All these diagnostic tests were performed at Eurofins Milk Testing Denmark, Vejen, Denmark, according to the manufacturer's instructions.

Nasal swabs from cows and calves and tracheal washes from calves were tested for the presence of *M. bovis* using the Fluidigm PCR system at the Technical University of Denmark, Lyngby, Denmark, and a Ct value < 30 was considered positive [19]. Cutoff values and test performance have not yet been established for this test.

Table 1. Overview of the herd type and size, previous *Mycoplasma bovis*-associated disease history, as well as previous diagnostic test results (from 2012–2019) and results of additional samples taken (RC-Calves in 2019–2020) for *Mycoplasma bovis* classification of 12 Danish dairy cattle herds (RC = Robust calves project, N/A = not available, BTM = bulk tank milk).

Herd No.	Herd Type	No. of Cows [a]	PCR—Individual Cows [b] (Positives/n)	ELISA—Individual Cows/ Calves [c] (Positives/n)	BTM PCR [b] (Positives/n)	BTM ELISA [c] (Positives/n)	RC-Calves—ID Screen [d] (Positives/n)	RC-Calves—BioX 302 [c] (Positives/n)	RC-Calves—PCR Test [e] (Positives/n)	*Mycoplasma bovis* Disease Outbreak	*Mycoplasma bovis* Classification
1	RC	150	N/A	N/A	0/21	0/16	0/27	1/27	0/182	No [f]	Not infected
2	RC	190	0/348	N/A	0/14	0/8	0/27	2/27	1/209	No [f]	Not infected
3	RC	350	0/9	0/8	0/9	1/5	0/29	1/29	0/228	Yes (2013) [f]	Not infected
4	RC	220	0/1	N/A	0/10	0/6	0/29	0/29	0/172	No [f]	Not infected
5	RC	200	0/3	N/A	0/11	1/6	1/29	0/30	0/129	Yes (2012) [f]	Not infected
6	RC	700	1/398	N/A	0/9	2/5	16/30	2/30	3/431	No [f]	Infected within the last 5 years
7	RC	600	0/284	N/A	1/23	0/6	24/30	10/30	1/179	Yes (2014–2015) [f]	Infected within the last 5 years
8	Outbreak	190	7/140	85/372	0/34	0/23	N/A	N/A	N/A	Yes (2015–2016) [g]	Infected within the last 5 years
9	Outbreak	430	69/1188	70/282	18/327	1/9	N/A	N/A	N/A	Yes (2015–2016) [g]	Infected within the last 5 years
10	Outbreak	200	21/98	91/303	3/16	1/12	N/A	N/A	N/A	Yes (2015–2016) [g]	Infected within the last 5 years
11	RC	600	10/25	0/3	0/10	1/7	N/A	N/A	11/256	Yes (2014) [f]	Infected at sampling
12	RC	330	4/234	N/A	0/14	0/6	N/A	N/A	9/228	No [f]	Infected at sampling

[a] Average number of cows per year during 2016–2019 [b] Pathoproof Major-3 or Complete-16 assays (Thermo Scientific, Waltham, MA, USA) or Mastit 4 (DNA diagnostic, Risskov, Denmark), test results collected on the farmers' initiatives prior to this study (e.g., for herd health management), positive cycle threshold < 37 [c] BioX 302 (BioX Diagnostics, Rochefort, Belgium), test results collected on the farmers' initiatives prior to this study (e.g., for herd health management), positive ≥ 37 sample coefficient (ODC%) [d] ID screen® mycoplasma bovis indirect (IDvet, Grabels, France), positive ≥ 60 sample-to-positive percentage (S/P%) [e] Fluidigm In-house PCR (Technical University of Denmark), positive cycle threshold < 30. [f] According to the farmer [g] Confirmed test-positive for *M. bovis*.

4.4. Statistical Analysis

The correlation between serum and milk S/P% was calculated as the concordance correlation coefficient [23]. All data management and statistical analyses were carried out in R version 3.2.2 [24] using the packages "dplyr", "ggplot2", "gridExtra" and "DescTools".

5. Conclusions

In the present study, we gained and shared experience of using the ID screen for the detection of antibodies against *M. bovis* in adult dairy cows under field conditions and compared this with the results of the BioX 302 test. When using the ID screen, nearly all cows in all, but three non-infected herds tested positive, while in contrast, very few cows tested positive when using the BioX 302. The ID screen is therefore a much more sensitive test than the BioX 302. However, some herds without ongoing infection, and even some herds with no history of *M. bovis* infection also tested positive. This indicates either lack of specificity (e.g., cross-reactions with other mycoplasma species) or that the ID screen measures exposure to *M. bovis* rather than the colonization and dissemination of the organism in the infected animal. The latter implies that the interpretation and recommendations for using the ID screen should be different from that of BioX 302. A concordance correlation coefficient between the ID screen serum and milk results of 0.66 (95% CI: 0.58–0.72) indicates that easy-to-collect milk samples can replace serum samples for ID screen diagnosis of *M. bovis* in adult cows, and the use of ID screen on bulk tank milk samples for surveillance and control purposes is promising. This, in addition to assessments of the ID screen performance (in particular regarding the specificity) under field conditions can provide new research questions to pursue. We therefore recommend field studies for best practice diagnostic test evaluation of the ID screen.

Author Contributions: Conceptualization, M.B.P., L.P. and L.R.N.; methodology, M.B.P., L.P., L.M.P. and L.R.N.; R-code, M.B.P.; formal analysis, M.B.P.; resources, M.B.P., L.P., L.M.P. and L.R.N.; data curation, M.B.P., L.P., L.M.P. and L.R.N.; writing—original draft preparation, M.B.P.; writing—review & editing, M.B.P., L.P., L.M.P. and L.R.N.; visualization, M.B.P.; supervision, L.P. and L.R.N.; project administration, M.B.P., L.P. and L.R.N.; funding acquisition, M.B.P., L.P., L.M.P. and L.R.N. All authors have read and agreed to the published version of the manuscript.

Funding: This research was funded by "Foreningen KUSTOS af 1881" and the "Robuste kalve" project. Eurofins Milk Testing funded the ELISA tests and covered the laboratory costs.

Conflicts of Interest: The authors declare that they have no conflicts of interest. M.B.P. and L.R.N. were involved in the previous and ongoing research projects that this study builds on. L.P. is employed by SEGES, a farmers' organization carrying out research and innovation and offering advisory services for farmers. L.M.P. is employed by Eurofins Milk Testing Denmark, which offers commercial *Mycoplasma bovis* diagnostic testing for cattle farmers.

References

1. Nicholas, R.A.J.; Ayling, R.D. Mycoplasma bovis: Disease, diagnosis, and control. *Res. Vet. Sci.* **2003**, *74*, 105–112. [CrossRef]
2. Maunsell, F.P.; Donovan, G.A. Mycoplasma bovis Infections in young calves. *Vet. Clin. N. Am. Food Anim. Pract.* **2009**, *25*, 139–177. [CrossRef] [PubMed]
3. Maunsell, F.P.; Woolums, A.R.; Francoz, D.; Rosenbusch, R.F.; Step, D.L.; Wilson, D.J.; Janzen, E.D. Mycoplasma bovis Infections in Cattle. *J. Vet. Intern. Med.* **2011**, *25*, 772–783. [CrossRef] [PubMed]
4. Petersen, M.B. Mycoplasma Bovis in Dairy Cattle—Clinical Epidemiology and Antibody Measurements for Decision Making. Ph.D. Thesis, University of Copenhagen, Frederiksberg, Denmark, 15 August 2018.
5. Schibrowski, M.L.; Barnes, T.S.; Wawegama, N.K.; Vance, M.E.; Markham, P.F.; Mansell, P.D.; Marenda, M.S.; Kanci, A.; Perez-Casal, J.; Browning, G.F.; et al. The performance of three immune assays to assess the serological status of cattle experimentally exposed to Mycoplasma bovis. *Vet. Sci.* **2018**, *5*, 27. [CrossRef] [PubMed]
6. Wawegama, N.K.; Markham, P.F.; Kanci, A.; Schibrowski, M.; Oswin, S.; Barnes, T.S.; Firestone, S.M.; Mahony, T.J.; Browning, G.F. Evaluation of an IgG enzyme-linked immunosorbent assay as a serological assay for detection of mycoplasma bovis infection in feedlot cattle. *J. Clin. Microbiol.* **2016**, *54*, 1269–1275. [CrossRef] [PubMed]

7. Andersson, A.M.; Aspán, A.; Wisselink, H.J.; Smid, B.; Ridley, A.; Pelkonen, S.; Autio, T.; Lauritsen, K.T.; Kensø, J.; Gaurivaud, P.; et al. A European inter-laboratory trial to evaluate the performance of three serological methods for diagnosis of Mycoplasma bovis infection in cattle using latent class analysis. *BMC Vet. Res.* **2019**, *15*, 1–10. [CrossRef] [PubMed]
8. Petersen, M.B.; Pedersen, J.; Holm, D.L.; Denwood, M.; Nielsen, L.R. A longitudinal observational study of the dynamics of Mycoplasma bovis antibodies in naturally exposed and diseased dairy cows. *J. Dairy Sci.* **2018**, *101*, 7386–7396. [CrossRef] [PubMed]
9. Petersen, M.B.; Wawegama, N.K.; Denwood, M.; Markham, P.F.; Browning, G.F.; Nielsen, L.R. Mycoplasma bovis antibody dynamics in naturally exposed dairy calves according to two diagnostic tests. *BMC Vet. Res.* **2018**, *14*. [CrossRef]
10. Bürki, S.; Frey, J.; Pilo, P. Virulence, persistence and dissemination of Mycoplasma bovis. *Vet. Microbiol.* **2015**, *179*, 15–22. [CrossRef]
11. Vähänikkilä, N.; Pohjanvirta, T.; Haapala, V.; Simojoki, H.; Soveri, T.; Browning, G.F.; Pelkonen, S.; Wawegama, N.K.; Autio, T. Characterisation of the course of Mycoplasma bovis infection in naturally infected dairy herds. *Vet. Microbiol.* **2019**, *231*, 107–115. [CrossRef] [PubMed]
12. Anonymous. Internal Validation Report ID Screen®Mycoplasma Bovis Indirect. Available online: https://www.id-vet.com/produit/id-screen-mycoplasma-bovis-indirect/ (accessed on 30 June 2020).
13. Howard, C.J.; Gourlay, R.N. Imunne Response Of Calves Following The Inoculation Of Mycoplasma Dispar And Mycoplasma Bovis. *Vet. Microbiol.* **1983**, *8*, 45–56. [CrossRef]
14. Jacobson, R.H. Validation of serological assays for diagnosis of infectious diseases. *Rev. Sci. et Tech. de l'OIE* **1998**, *17*, 469–486. [CrossRef] [PubMed]
15. Nielsen, P.K.; Petersen, M.B.; Nielsen, L.R.; Halasa, T.; Toft, N. Latent class analysis of bulk tank milk PCR and ELISA testing for herd level diagnosis of Mycoplasma bovis. *Prev. Vet. Med.* **2015**, *121*, 338–342. [CrossRef] [PubMed]
16. Parker, A.M.; House, J.K.; Hazelton, M.S.; Bosward, K.L.; Morton, J.M.; Sheehy, P.A. Bulk tank milk antibody ELISA as a biosecurity tool for detecting dairy herds with past exposure to Mycoplasma bovis. *J. Dairy Sci.* **2017**, *100*, 8296–8309. [CrossRef] [PubMed]
17. Anonymous. Standard Operating Procedure for OIE Registration of Diagnostic Kits. Available online: https://www.oie.int/doc/ged/D12069.PDF (accessed on 29 July 2020).
18. Petersen, M.B.; Krogh, K.; Nielsen, L.R. Factors associated with variation in bulk tank milk Mycoplasma bovis antibody-ELISA results in dairy herds. *J. Dairy Sci.* **2016**, *99*, 3815–3823. [CrossRef] [PubMed]
19. Goecke, N.B.; Hjulsager, C.K.; Krog, J.S.; Skovgaard, K.; Larsen, L.E. Development of a high-throughput real-time PCR system for detection of enzootic pathogens in pigs. *J. Vet. Diagn. Investig.* **2020**, *32*, 51–64. [CrossRef] [PubMed]
20. Wawegama, N.K.; Browning, G.F.; Kanci, A.; Marenda, M.S.; Markham, P.F. Development of a recombinant protein-based enzyme-linked immunosorbent assay for diagnosis of mycoplasma bovis infection in cattle. *Clin. Vaccine Immunol.* **2014**, *21*, 196–202. [CrossRef] [PubMed]
21. Anonymous. IDVet Screen Mycoplasma Bovis Indirect Material Safety Data Sheet. Available online: https://www.id-vet.com/produit/id-screen-mycoplasma-bovis-indirect/ (accessed on 30 June 2020).
22. Anonymous. BioX Diagnostics Monoscreen Ab ELISA. Available online: https://www.biox.com/en/bio-k-302-monoscreen-abelisa-mycoplasma-bovis-indirect-monowell-p-250/ (accessed on 30 June 2020).
23. Lin, L.I.-K. A Concordance Correlation Coefficient to Evaluate Reproducibility. *Biometrics* **1989**, *45*, 255. [CrossRef] [PubMed]
24. R Core Team. R: A Language and Environment for Statistical Computing. R Foundation for Statistical Computing: Vienna, Austria,2016. Available online: https://www.R-project.org/ (accessed on 30 June 2020).

pathogens

MDPI

Article

Infection Dynamics of *Mycoplasma bovis* and Other Respiratory Mycoplasmas in Newly Imported Bulls on Italian Fattening Farms

Salvatore Catania [1], Michele Gastaldelli [1], Eliana Schiavon [1], Andrea Matucci [1], Annalucia Tondo [1], Marianna Merenda [1] and Robin A. J. Nicholas [2,*]

1 Istituto Zooprofilattico Sperimentale delle Venezie, viale Dell'Università 10, 371735 Legnaro, PD, Italy; scatania@izsvenezie.it (S.C.); mgastaldelli@izsvenezie.it (M.G.); eschiavon@izsvenezie.it (E.S.); amatucci@izsvenezie.it (A.M.); atondo@izsvenezie.it (A.T.); mmerenda@izsvenezie.it (M.M.)

2 The Oaks, Nutshell Lane, Farnham, Surrey GU9 0HG, UK

* Correspondence: robin.a.j.nicholas@gmail.com; Tel.: +44-1252-725557

Received: 3 June 2020; Accepted: 29 June 2020; Published: 4 July 2020

Abstract: Italian beef production is mainly based on a feedlot system where calves are housed with mixed aged cattle often in conditions favourable to bovine respiratory disease (BRD). In Veneto, an indoor system is also used for imported bulls around 300–350 kg. Mycoplasmas, in particular *Mycoplasma bovis* and *Mycoplasma dispar*, contribute to BRD in young calves, but their role in the disease in older cattle has not been investigated. In this study, ten heads of cattle were selected from each of the 24 groups kept in 13 different farms. Bulls were sampled by nasal swabbing at 0, 15, and 60 days after arrival for *Mycoplasma* isolation. Identification was carried out by 16S-rDNA PCR followed by denaturing gradient gel electrophoresis. *M. bovis*, *M. dispar*, and *M. bovirhinis* were identified, and prevalence was analysed by mixed-effects logistic regression models. This showed that most bulls arrived free of *M. bovis*, but within two weeks, approximately 40% became infected, decreasing to 13% by the last sampling. In contrast, the prevalence of *M. dispar* was not dependent on time or seasonality, while *M. bovirhinis* only showed a seasonality-dependent trend. The Italian fattening system creates an ideal environment for infection with *M. bovis*, probably originating from previously stabled animals.

Keywords: *Mycoplasma bovis*; bovine respiratory disease; cattle; prevalence

1. Introduction

Most European countries operate a feedlot system for male beef production where young calves, usually about one month old, are brought in mostly from dairy farms, then fattened to approximately 240 kg. In Italy, a mixed-age indoor system is also used, which involves the importation of bulls at 300–350 kg from other European countries. This system is mainly located in the Po Valley with the largest herds in the Veneto region [1] and accounts for approximately an 85% share of the beef market. On arrival, the bulls are placed indoors directly with cattle of different ages often sharing the same air space. The cattle are kept for approximately 6 months until they reach a target weight of approximately 650 kg. While relatively productive, the system is prone to severe outbreaks of bovine respiratory disease (BRD) caused by different pathogens, such as bovine viral diarrhoea (BVD) virus, para-influenza virus 3 (PI3), infectious bovine rhinotracheitis (IBR) virus, *Pasteurella*, *Mannheimia*, and mycoplasmas [2]. BRD is often exacerbated by overcrowding and poor ventilation and compounded by the heterogeneity of breeds and diverse origins of the cattle.

At least 30 different mycoplasmas have been isolated from cattle, of which only a few are considered pathogenic, notably *Mycoplasma bovis* and *M. dispar*, which can cause serious respiratory disease in young and adult animals, respectively [3]. Other mycoplasmas have a pathogenic impact on the reproductive system, such as *M. bovigenitalium* [4], while others, such as *M. bovis, M. californicum,* and *M. canadense,* are causes of or associated with mastitis [5]. *M. bovirhinis* is frequently isolated from the respiratory tract but is mostly considered to be non-pathogenic [6].

M. bovis has been identified as the major pathogen affecting young animals in northern Italy [2] and is suspected of being involved in disease in older livestock. For this reason, we decided to investigate the prevalence and epidemiology of *Mycoplasma* species in this specialised older cattle sector.

In this study, we used *Mycoplasma* isolation and species identification by 16S-rDNA PCR, followed by denaturing gradient gel electrophoresis (DGGE) to assess the prevalence of *M. bovis, M. dispar,* and *M. bovirhinis* in different batches of imported bulls stabled in Italian farms. Animals were sampled by nasal swabs at different times after arrival following a longitudinal experimental design. In addition to isolation, *M. bovis* presence was also determined by a specific PCR protocol.

2. Results

Of the 711 analysed nasal swabs, 485 (68.2%) were positive for species belonging to the *Mollicutes* class. The majority of the isolated organisms belonged to the species *M. bovirhinis* (283, 39.8%), *M. bovis* (136, 19.1%), *M. dispar* (86, 12.1%), and to species of the genus *Ureaplasma* (66, 9.3%) (Table S1). Approximately half of all isolated organisms were found in mixed cultures with other species of the *Mollicutes* class. In addition, *M. bovis* was detected in 276 swabs (approximately 39% of the total samples) by direct PCR in contrast to the 136 isolates (19% of the total samples) obtained by culture.

2.1. Analysis of Prevalence of Mollicutes Class Organisms

Isolates identified as belonging to the *Mollicutes* class largely varied in prevalence over time post-arrival and among the different bull batches and fattening farms (Figure 1a).

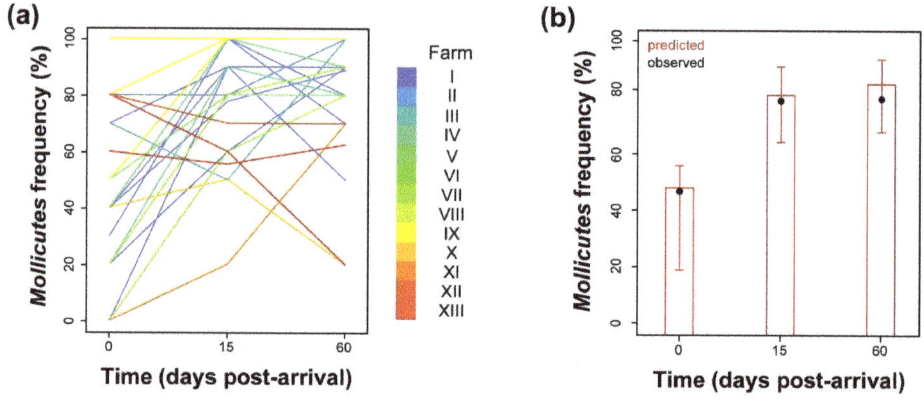

Figure 1. (**a**) Batch-related frequency of isolation of organisms belonging to the *Mollicutes* class analysed over time after arrival. Each line colour is depicted according to the identity of the stabling farm. (**b**) Model-predicted *Mollicutes* prevalence inferred at the population level over time post arrival (red). Observed mean prevalence values are depicted as solid black circles. Vertical lines correspond to the 95% CI of the predicted mean.

However, at the population level, we could identify a clear, significant time-dependent trend (Tables S2 and S3) characterised by an initial prevalence value of incoming animals of approximately 48%, with a 95% confidence interval (95% CI) ranging from 30% to 67%. At 15 days post-arrival (p.a.), the estimated frequency of *Mollicutes*-positive animals significantly increased with an odds ratio of 4.6 (95% CI, 2.2–10.5; adjusted $p = 0.003$) to reach a plateau at approximately 81% (Figure 1b). No effects of the environmental conditions (variable "season", see the paragraph in Materials and Methods) on predicted prevalence were observed (Table S3).

2.2. Analysis of Prevalence of *M. bovis*

The frequency of *M. bovis* isolation clearly varied in a time-dependent fashion (Figure 2a). At arrival, 18 of 24 batches (75%) were negative for *M. bovis*, and 21 (87.5%) showed a prevalence lower than 10%. Such results were confirmed by PCR (Figure 2b): 17 of 24 batches (71%) were negative at arrival, and 20 (83%) showed a prevalence lower than 10%.

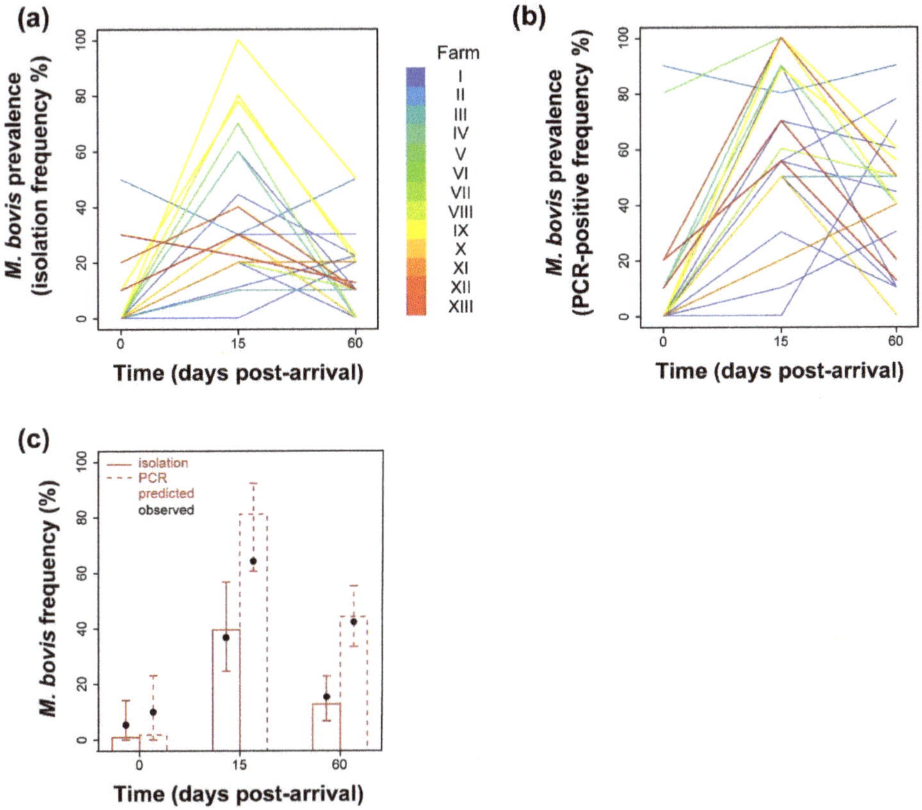

Figure 2. (**a**) Batch-related frequency of isolation of *M. bovis* analysed over time after arrival. Each line colour is depicted according to the identity of the stabling farm. (**b**) Batch-related frequency of *M. bovis*-specific PCR positives among bull batches analysed over time after arrival. (**c**) Model-predicted *M. bovis* prevalence, inferred at the population level and assessed from isolation (continuous line) and PCR (dashed line) data. Observed mean prevalence values from isolation and PCR data are depicted as solid black circles. Vertical lines correspond to the 95% CI of the predicted mean.

With both approaches, we could clearly observe an increase in frequency at 15 p.a., followed by a general decrease 45 days later, which however largely varied in rate among farms/batches. The logistic models constructed confirmed such observations (Tables S4 and S6). At the population level, the probability of isolating *M. bovis* or testing bulls positive by PCR significantly depended on the time of sampling (Tables S5 and S7). The mean predicted *M. bovis* prevalence among newly introduced animals was estimated in the range of 1–2%, with upper confidence limits of 14% (isolation) and 23% (PCR) (Figure 2c). Such prevalence dramatically increased 15 days after introduction into stables, with an odds ratio of 73.4 for isolation (95% CI, 6.7–750, adjusted $p = 0.015$) and 213 for PCR (95% CI, 35–1901, adjusted $p = 0.0001$), to reach an estimated prevalence of approximately 40% (95% CI, 25–57%) in case of isolation and 81% (95% CI, 61–92%) according to PCR. At 60 days p.a., the estimated prevalence dropped to a lower level that differed with respect to the preceding one only when considering PCR-based frequency (adjusted $p = 0.02$). Environmental conditions did not show any predictive role in *M. bovis* prevalence (Tables S5 and S7).

2.3. Analysis of Prevalence of *M. dispar*

Unlike *M. bovis*, the analysis of prevalence of *M. dispar* did not show any dependence on time, as shown by the batch trend lines (Figure 3) and the model we constructed (Tables S8 and S9). In fact, the mean predicted prevalence was estimated as constant with a value of 9.4% (95% CI, 6.7—13%). Similar to time, inclusion of seasonality did not increase the predictive power of the model (Table S9).

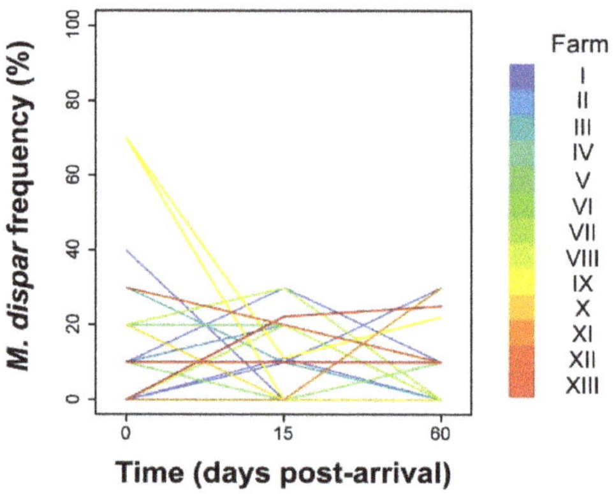

Figure 3. Batch-related frequency of isolation of *M. dispar* analysed over time after arrival. Each line colour is depicted according to the identity of the stabling farm.

2.4. Analysis of Prevalence of *M. bovirhinis*

As already observed especially in the case of *M. bovis*, trend analysis of *M. bovirhinis* isolation over time post-arrival showed high variability among the sampled batches/farms (Figure 4a). Although there appeared to be an increase in prevalence over time, this was not significant (Table S11). Instead, we found that *M. bovirhinis* isolation probability depended on the stabling environmental conditions described by the variable "season" (Tables S10 and S11). In fact, the estimated mean prevalence of *M. bovirhinis* passed from 21.6% (95% CI, 12.9–33.9%), observed in the cold months of the year, to 33.1% (95% CI, 20–49.4%) in the warm season (Figure 4b), with an odds ratio of 1.8 (95% CI, 1.08–2.77).

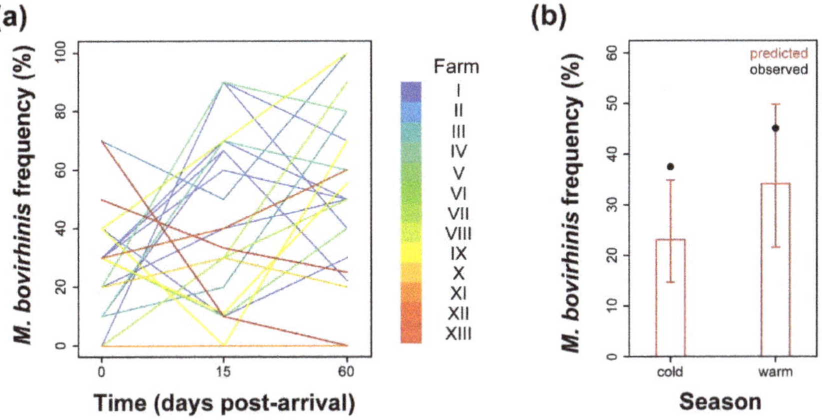

Figure 4. (**a**) Batch-related frequency of isolation of *M. bovirhinis* analysed over time after arrival. Each line colour is depicted according to the identity of the stabling farm. (**b**) Model-predicted *M. bovirhinis* prevalence inferred at the population level over arrival season (red). Observed mean prevalence values are depicted as solid black circles. Vertical lines correspond to the 95% CI of the predicted mean.

3. Discussion

The impact of BRD on cattle production is estimated to cause a decrease in mean carcass weight of at least 9 kg, leading to heavy losses of farmers' incomes [7]. A better understanding of the spread of bovine mycoplasmas, involved in the BRD complex, may thus benefit practitioners by providing them with more comprehensive advice on how to control this significant economic and welfare problem [8]. The Italian bull production system is based on a singular approach typical of northeastern Italy and is believed, by local practitioners, to be exceptionally susceptible to BRD with a significant role played by mycoplasmas. However, the problems of this type of farming have not been well studied, leading to a poor understanding of the causes and risk factors of BRD.

The results of the present study showed that most nasal samples taken from bulls throughout the testing period were positive for organisms belonging to the *Mollicutes* class. Amplification of a fragment of the 16s rRNA gene followed by DGGE and profile comparison with reference strains led to their identification at species level (Table S1). In 71% of the cases, swabs were positive to *M. bovis* (19.1%), *M. dispar* (12.1%), and/or *M. bovirhinis* (39.8%) species, as pure or mixed cultures. In a previous work on Danish cattle farms [9], similar proportions of *M. bovirhinis* and *M. dispar* were detected, but *M bovis* was surprisingly absent. Our results showed a significant presence of *M. bovis* in the Italian bull meat sector with nearly a fifth of samples being positive, confirming other reports on the high prevalence of this mycoplasma in Britain [6], Ireland [10], France [8], and Canada [11].

In the present study, it appears evident that the majority of bulls arrived at the farm free of *M. bovis*, but within 2 weeks, its prevalence dramatically increased up to approximately 40% and 81% when tested by culture and *M. bovis*-specific PCR, respectively. Although high variability was observed at farm/batch level, our results showed that there was a rapid spread of *M. bovis* to the newly arrived bulls most likely from infected cattle already on the farm and/or possibly from the small number of infected imported bulls. In this regard, the phylogenetical typing of isolated strains could be useful to better understand the mechanism whereby *M. bovis* spreads among imported bulls, and future studies on that are strongly advised. The decrease in the percentage of infected cattle at 60 days p.a. indicates that some bulls overcame the infection to a point where it was no longer detectable in individual animals probably as a result of the host immune response mounted against this pathogen. Such a trend was seen in whatever diagnostic method used to detect *M. bovis*-positive bulls.

In contrast to *M. bovis*, *M. dispar* prevalence did not follow a time-dependent behaviour. Much variability was observed among batches and farms (Figure 3), such that at the population level, it did not allow to reveal a common, statistically significant trend, suggesting a constant prevalence of 9.4%. Similarly, stabling animals in different seasons did not change the rate of spread of *M. dispar*. General unfavourable environmental conditions and/or the specific immune status of the bulls may account for the observed differences in the rate of spread between *M. bovis* and *M. dispar*. In our opinion, the low prevalence of *M. bovis* among incoming animals suggests the majority of these individuals may have been naïve to *M. bovis* infection, a condition that facilitated the spread of farm-resident *M. bovis* strains, exacerbated by the close contact with infected older bulls in overcrowded conditions. In contrast, the higher *M. dispar* prevalence observed already on arrival may indicate that the immune systems of the incoming animals were already primed to this mycoplasma species, providing a protective shield against *M. dispar* infection and spread. Alternatively, an unfavourable environment and breeding conditions may have limited the spread. It is also possible that the high prevalence of *M. bovis* may have competitively excluded the colonisation of *M dispar* although evidence is needed to support this.

Similarly to *M. dispar*, *M. bovirhinis* prevalence showed high variability among batches and farms, such that we could not statistically define a common trend over time. However, we observed a significant effect of environmental conditions brought about by seasonality, with higher prevalence associated with warmer conditions. This trait seems to be specific for this species as it was not observed with *M. bovis* and *M. dispar*. *M. bovirhinis* is not considered a primary pathogen and, although it is one of the most commonly occurring species in respiratory diseases [6], it can also be frequently isolated from healthy or asymptomatic animals, where it may be considered part of the natural bacterial flora. The decrease in prevalence of *M. bovirhinis* seen in the winter months may be due to the preferential colonisation of respiratory pathogens, including *M. bovis* and *M. dispar* [12–14], when cattle are more susceptible. Alternatively, such an association may derive from spurious effects given by hidden confounding variables.

In conclusion, our results showed that the Italian fattening bull system creates an ideal environment for the spread and diffusion of *Mollicutes* and, more specifically, of *M. bovis*. The spread of the latter did not seem to be related to the health status of the new bulls; in fact, the high circulation of *M. bovis* is localised during the first weeks after arrival. Most likely, the spread was related to the presence of older infected bulls that provided the source of infection, possibly a dominant farm-specific *M. bovis* strain, to the newly imported bulls as previously reported [8]. A similar situation is seen in other livestock sectors, such as multiage layers hens flocks where the spread of mycoplasma from older birds can cause economic losses in the newest flocks [15,16]. This kind of problem has been controlled in the poultry industry by "all in, all out" systems stocked with *Mycoplasma*-free or by vaccination and could be applied with specific modifications to the bull meat sector studied here. The newly acquired knowledge of *M. bovis* diffusion dynamics from this study will enable better management of BRD, focusing on the herd management, such as improving ventilation and other husbandry techniques.

4. Materials and Methods

4.1. Animals

In this study, we longitudinally analysed 24 different male cattle batches, imported in 2011–2013 and stabled into 13 different fattening farms (identified as I–XIII) of Northern Italy. Most batches consisted of 54 heads of cattle, in large part imported from France. The capacity of the selected farms differed among each other, ranging from 400 to 1500 bulls per farm. For each batch, 10 bulls were randomly selected and sampled for the entire period of the study, with the exception of 7 animals that were lost during the observational period due to mortality or slaughtering (Table S12). Two deep nasal swabs, one for *M. bovis* PCR and the other for *Mollicutes* isolation, were taken from each animal on arrival, and at 15 and 60 days after arrival. A total of 711 samples were collected: 240 on arrival, 238 at the second, and 233 at the third sampling.

4.2. Mollicute Cultivation

To ensure *Mollicutes* vitality, immediately after sampling, swabs were immersed into 2 mL of *Mycoplasma* liquid medium (ML; Mycoplasma Experience Ltd., Bletchingley, UK) and maintained at 4 °C until arrival at the laboratory. Mycoplasma cultivation and isolation were then performed in ML and PPLO (Pleuro-Pneumonia like Organisms) broth media. Briefly, the inoculated cultures were incubated at 37 °C with 5% CO_2 for at least 7 days. The broths were checked daily up to 14 days to detect any change in colour or turbidity. Broths that showed any change were immediately inoculated onto a plate of semisolid *Mycoplasma* agar medium (MS; Mycoplasma Experience). Alternatively, broths that did not show any change were plated onto agar medium at the end of the observation period. If no colonies grew after 14 days, the sample was considered negative.

4.3. Mycoplasma Identification

To identify the species of the different *Mollicutes* grown in broth media, DNA was extracted with the Maxwell 16 LEV Blood DNA kit and Maxwell 16 Instrument following the manufacturer's instructions (Promega), amplified by a 16S-rDNA-targeting PCR and analysed by denaturing gradient gel electrophoresis (DGGE), following a previously reported protocol [17]. Identification of the different *Mollicutes* genera and species was carried out by direct comparison of the lane of interest with the profile of reference strains. To investigate the presence of *M. bovis* DNA on the collected swabs, total DNA was extracted from an aliquot of the relative transport medium, amplified by a *M. bovis*-specific PCR protocol [18] and analysed by electrophoresis in 1% agar gel.

4.4. Statistical Analysis

The statistical analysis of this study was conducted under R environment [19]. The prevalence of organisms belonging to the *Mollicutes* class and to the species *M. bovis*, *M. dispar*, and *M. bovirhinis* was analysed according to a longitudinal framework, in which the same animals were repeatedly sampled along time post arrival. In addition, the potential correlation among observations from the same animals (coded by the variable "ID") and from bulls belonging to the same batch ("batch" variable) or farm ("farm" variable) was considered. For such reasons, we decided to construct logistic mixed effects (hierarchical) models to predict bulls' positivity to each of the 4 considered organisms. For all models, we first determined the correlation structure that best suited to the observed data. Random intercept models were constructed, assuming as random effects the covariates "ID", "farm", and "batch" alone or in nestling combinations. Random intercept and slope models were then evaluated, adding a random slope described by the categorical covariate "time" (time post arrival) to the previously selected random intercept model. In all cases, the best-fitting correlation structure was described by a random slope associated to the covariate "time" and a random intercept expressed by the grouping variable "farm". At the population level, in addition to the covariate "time", we tested the descriptive variable "season", coded as "cold" if the bulls were stabled between November and March and "warm" otherwise. The significance of both random and fixed effects variables was estimated by repeated likelihood ratio tests. All models but the ones predicting the probability of isolating *M. bovis* and *M. dispar* were estimated with the function *glmer* of the *lme4* package [20], applying a maximum likelihood with Laplace approximation and "bobyqa" optimisation for convergence. In the case of the models describing *M. bovis* and *M. dispar* prevalence from isolation, the aforementioned approach led to singular fits, in which some components of the variance–covariance matrix were estimated as zero. To overcome this problem, we employed the function *bglmer* of the package *blme* [21] that allows obtaining inferences based on a penalised maximum likelihood with priors for the covariance matrix of the random effects following a Wishart distribution. Multiple comparisons were performed with the function *pairs* of the package *emmeans*, applying Tukey's p value adjustment method [22].

Supplementary Materials: The following are available online at http://www.mdpi.com/2076-0817/9/7/537/s1, Table S1: Species and genera of the *Mollicutes* class isolated from the analysed nasal swabs. Table S2: Parameter estimates of the logistic mixed effects model analysing the isolation frequency of organisms of the *Mollicutes* class. Table S3: Analysis of deviance table (type II likelihood ratio tests) of the full model relating the isolation frequency of organisms of the *Mollicutes* class to the variables time and season.. Table S4: Parameter estimates of the logistic mixed effects model analyzing the frequency of *M. bovis* isolation. Table S5: Analysis of deviance table (type II likelihood ratio tests) of the full model relating the frequency of isolation of *M. bovis* to the variables time and season. Table S6: Parameter estimates of the logistic mixed effects model analyzing the frequency of *M. bovis*-specific PCR positives. Table S7: Analysis of deviance table (type II likelihood ratio tests) of the full model relating the frequency of *M. bovis*-specific PCR positives to the variables time and season. Table S8: Parameter estimates of the logistic mixed effects model analyzing the frequency of *M. dispar* isolation. Table S9: Analysis of deviance table (type II likelihood ratio tests) of the full model relating the frequency of isolation of *M. dispar* to the variables time and season. Table S10: Parameter estimates of the logistic mixed effects model analyzing the frequency of *M. bovirhinis* isolation. Table S11: Analysis of deviance table (type II likelihood ratio tests) of the full model relating the frequency of isolation of *M. bovirhinis* to the variables time and season. Table S12: Data structure description.

Author Contributions: Conceptualisation, S.C. and R.A.J.N.; *Mollicute* cultivation and identification, A.M. and A.T.; software, M.G.; formal analysis, M.G.; investigation, E.S. and M.M.; data curation, S.C., M.M., and M.G.; writing—original draft preparation, S.C.; writing—review and editing, M.G. and R.A.J.N.; visualisation, M.G.; supervision, S.C. and R.A.J.N.; project administration, S.C. and R.A.J.N.; funding acquisition, S.C. and R.A.J.N. All authors have read and agreed to the published version of the manuscript.

Funding: This research received no external funding.

Conflicts of Interest: The authors declare no conflict of interest.

References

1. Cozzi, G. Present situation and future challenges of beef cattle production in Italy and the role of the research. *Ital. J. Anim. Sci.* **2007**, *6* (Suppl. 1), 389–396. [CrossRef]
2. Radaelli, E.; Luini, M.; Loria, G.R.; Nicholas, R.A.J.; Scanziani, E. Bacteriological, serological, pathological and immunohistochemical studies of *Mycoplasma bovis* respiratory infection in veal calves and adult cattle at slaughter. *Res. Vet. Sci.* **2008**, *85*, 282–290. [CrossRef] [PubMed]
3. Nicholas, R.A.J.; Ayling, R.D. *Mycoplasma bovis*: Disease, diagnosis, and control. *Res. Vet. Sci.* **2003**, *74*, 105–112. [CrossRef]
4. Nicholas, R.; Ayling, R.; McAuliffe, L. *Mycoplasma Diseases of Ruminants*; CABI Publishing: Wallingford, UK, 2008; ISBN 9780851990125.
5. Nicholas, R.A.J.; Fox, L.K.; Lysnyansky, I. Mycoplasma mastitis in cattle: To cull or not to cull. *Vet. J.* **2016**, *216*, 142–147. [CrossRef] [PubMed]
6. Ayling, R.D.; Bashiruddin, S.E.; Nicholas, R.A.J. *Mycoplasma* species and related organisms isolated from ruminants in Britain between 1990 and 2000. *Vet. Rec.* **2004**, *155*, 413–416. [CrossRef] [PubMed]
7. Pardon, B.; Hostens, M.; Duchateau, L.; Dewulf, J.; De Bleecker, K.; Deprez, P. Impact of respiratory disease, diarrhea, otitis and arthritis on mortality and carcass traits in white veal calves. *BMC Vet. Res.* **2013**, *9*, 79. [CrossRef] [PubMed]
8. Timsit, E.; Arcangioli, M.-A.; Bareille, N.; Seegers, H.; Assié, S. Transmission dynamics of *Mycoplasma bovis* in newly received beef bulls at fattening operations. *J. Vet. Diagn. Investig.* **2012**, *24*, 1172–1176. [CrossRef] [PubMed]
9. Angen, Ø.; Thomsen, J.; Larsen, L.E.; Larsen, J.; Kokotovic, B.; Heegaard, P.M.H.; Enemark, J.M.D. Respiratory disease in calves: Microbiological investigations on trans-tracheally aspirated bronchoalveolar fluid and acute phase protein response. *Vet. Microbiol.* **2009**, *137*, 165–171. [CrossRef] [PubMed]
10. Bell, C.J.; Blackburn, P.; Elliott, M.; Patterson, T.I.A.P.; Ellison, S.; Lahuerta-Marin, A.; Ball, H.J. Investigation of polymerase chain reaction assays to improve detection of bacterial involvement in bovine respiratory disease. *J. Vet. Diagn. Investig.* **2014**, *26*, 631–634. [CrossRef] [PubMed]
11. Booker, C.W.; Abutarbush, S.M.; Morley, P.S.; Jim, G.K.; Pittman, T.J.; Schunicht, O.C.; Perrett, T.; Wildman, B.K.; Fenton, R.K.; Guichon, P.T.; et al. Microbiological and histopathological findings in cases of fatal bovine respiratory disease of feedlot cattle in western Canada. *Can. Vet. J.* **2008**, *49*, 473. [PubMed]
12. O'Neill, R.; Mooney, J.; Connaghan, E.; Furphy, C.; Graham, D.A. Patterns of detection of respiratory viruses in nasal swabs from calves in Ireland: A retrospective study. *Vet. Rec.* **2014**, *175*, 35. [CrossRef] [PubMed]

13. Stein, R.A.; Katz, D.E. Escherichia coli, cattle and the propagation of disease. *FEMS Microbiol. Lett.* **2017**, *364*, 1–11. [CrossRef]
14. Abdelhay Kaoud, H. Introductory Chapter: Bacterial Cattle Diseases—Economic Impact and Their Control. In *Bacterial Cattle Diseases*; IntechOpen: London, UK, 2019.
15. Catania, S.; Gobbo, F.; Bilato, D.; Gagliazzo, L.; Moronato, M.L.; Terregino, C.; Bradbury, J.M.; Ramírez, A.S. Two strains of Mycoplasma synoviae from chicken flocks on the same layer farm differ in their ability to produce eggshell apex abnormality. *Vet. Microbiol.* **2016**, *193*, 60–66. [CrossRef] [PubMed]
16. Catania, S.; Bilato, D.; Gobbo, F.; Granato, A.; Terregino, C.; Iob, L.; Nicholas, R.A.J. Treatment of Eggshell Abnormalities and Reduced Egg Production Caused by Mycoplasma synoviae Infection. *Avian Dis.* **2010**, *54*, 961–964. [CrossRef] [PubMed]
17. McAuliffe, L.; Ellis, R.J.; Lawes, J.R.; Ayling, R.D.; Nicholas, R.A.J. 16S rDNA PCR and denaturing gradient gel electrophoresis; a single generic test for detecting and differentiating Mycoplasma species. *J. Med. Microbiol.* **2005**, *54*, 731–739. [CrossRef] [PubMed]
18. Butler, J.A.; Pinnow, C.C.; Thomson, J.U.; Levisohn, S.; Rosenbusch, R.F. Use of arbitrarily primed polymerase chain reaction to investigate Mycoplasma bovis outbreaks. *Vet. Microbiol.* **2001**, *78*, 175–181. [CrossRef]
19. R Core Team. *R: A Language and Environment for Statistical Computing 2019*; R Foundation for Statistical Computing: Vienna, Austria; Available online: https://www.R-project.org/ (accessed on 1 July 2020).
20. Bates, D.; Mächler, M.; Bolker, B.; Walker, S. Fitting Linear Mixed-Effects Models Using {lme4}. *J. Stat. Softw.* **2015**, *67*, 1–48. [CrossRef]
21. Chung, Y.; Rabe-Hesketh, S.; Dorie, V.; Gelman, A.; Liu, J. A nondegenerate penalized likelihood estimator for variance parameters in multilevel models. *Psychometrika* **2013**, *78*, 685–709. [CrossRef] [PubMed]
22. Lenth, R. Emmeans: Estimated Marginal Means, Aka Least-Squares Means. R Package Version 1.4.6. 2019. Available online: https://CRAN.R-project.org/package=emmean (accessed on 1 July 2020).

pathogens

MDPI

Article

Efficacy of Two Antibiotic-Extender Combinations on *Mycoplasma bovis* in Bovine Semen Production

Tarja Pohjanvirta [1,*], Nella Vähänikkilä [1], Henri Simonen [2], Sinikka Pelkonen [1] and Tiina Autio [1]

[1] Finnish Food Authority, Laboratory and Research Division, Veterinary Bacteriology and Pathology Unit, Neulaniementie 4, 70210 Kuopio, Finland; nella.vahanikkila@foodauthority.fi (N.V.); sinikka.pelkonen@foodauthority.fi (S.P.); tiina.autio@foodauthority.fi (T.A.)

[2] VikingGenetics, Korpikyläntie 77, 15870 Hollola, Finland; hesim@vikinggenetics.com

* Correspondence: tarja.pohjanvirta@foodauthority.fi; Tel.: +358-447-201-493

Received: 21 August 2020; Accepted: 29 September 2020; Published: 30 September 2020

Abstract: *Mycoplasma bovis* is an important bovine pathogen. Artificial insemination (AI) using contaminated semen can introduce the agent into a naïve herd. Antibiotics, most often gentamycin, tylosin, lincomycin, spectinomycin (GTLS) combination are added to semen extender to prevent transmission of pathogenic bacteria and mycoplasmas. In a commercial AI straw production system with industrial scale procedures, we analyzed the mycoplasmacidal efficacy of GTLS and ofloxacin on *M. bovis* ATCC and wild type strain isolated from commercial AI straws. The strains were spiked at two concentrations (10^6 and 10^3 CFU/mL) into semen. Viable *M. bovis* in frozen semen straws was detected by enrichment culture and real-time PCR. We also compared different protocols to extract *M. bovis* DNA from spiked semen. None of the antibiotic protocols had any effect on the viability of either of the *M. bovis* strains at high spiking concentration. At low concentration, the wild type was inhibited by all other protocols, except low GTLS, whereas the ATCC strain was inhibited only by high GTLS. The InstaGene™ matrix was the most effective method to extract *M. bovis* DNA from semen. When there is a low *M. bovis* contamination level in semen, GTLS used at high concentrations, in accordance with Certified Semen Services requirements, is more efficient than GTLS used at concentrations stated in the OIE Terrestrial Code.

Keywords: *Mycoplasma bovis*; bovine semen; antibiotics; prevention; DNA extraction

1. Introduction

Mycoplasma bovis is a major bovine pathogen causing substantial economic losses and has a debilitating effect on animal welfare. *M. bovis* causes a variety of diseases including mastitis, pneumonia, arthritis, otitis media, and genital infections [1]. Efforts to develop efficacious vaccines have not been successful [2]. Once established in a cattle farm, *M. bovis* can be difficult to eradicate [3]. Consequently, it is of paramount importance to prevent the introduction of the agent into naïve herds.

One *M. bovis* transmission route into a herd is artificial insemination (AI) [4]. Recently, we reported on how contaminated semen used in AI, introduced *M. bovis* infection into closed naïve dairy herds [5]. In a previous study, heifers inseminated with semen containing *M. bovis* became repeat breeders, and only half of them finally conceived [6]. *M. bovis* could be isolated from cervico-vaginal mucus of some of the heifers, 8–32 weeks after insemination. Kissi et al. [7] showed that insemination with frozen *Mycoplasma sp.* containing semen often resulted in prolonged diestrus, suggesting that mycoplasma could initiate a pathological process in the uterus. However, very little is known about the concentration of *M. bovis* in naturally infected bull semen and the infectious dose needed to initiate an infection in the female genital system.

There are several viral and bacterial pathogens that can be transmitted via semen [8]. Semen used for AI should be free of infectious agents. Several types of antibiotics have been added to seminal extenders before freezing to control bacterial contamination, including mycoplasmas. The World Organization for Animal Health OIE lists, in the OIE Terrestrial Code [9], the following three different antibiotic combinations to be used in international trade of bovine semen: gentamicin (250 μg), tylosin (50 μg), lincomycin-spectinomycin (150/300 μg) (GTLS) in each mL of frozen semen; penicillin (500 IU), streptomycin (500 μg), lincomycin-spectinomycin (150/300 μg) (PSLS); or amikacin (75 μg), divekacin (25 μg). The European Union directive 88/407/1993 includes the use of the above mentioned PSLS, or an alternative combination of antibiotics with an equivalent effect against campylobacters, leptospires, and mycoplasmas. Shin et al. [10], in 1988, developed a method where GTLS concentration was doubled as compared with the concentration stated in OIE Code, and GTLS was first added into raw semen before extending with GTLS containing extender. Nowadays, GTLS is widely used in bovine semen production, and Certified Semen Services (CSS) in USA has a special protocol in place for GTLS use [11]. However, Visser et al. conducted two studies, in 1995 and 1999 [12,13], in which they questioned the ability of even the high GTLS concentration to control *M. bovis* in AI. Since the studies of Shin et al. [10] and Visser et al. [12,13], animal protein sources in commercial extenders have often been replaced with plant protein sources such as soybean lecithin to avoid disease transmission through the use of animal source protein [14]. Most commercially available soy-lecithin-based extenders contain GTLS as standard antibiotics. However, recent *M. bovis* isolates have shown a marked increase in MIC90 values for tylosin, lincomycin, and spectinomycin, but resistance against fluoroquinolones is still quite rare [15–17]. Recently a fluoroquinolone antibiotic, ofloxacin, was shown to be non-toxic to spermatozoa and effective in protecting semen from bacteria, although the authors did not analyze its effect on mycoplasmas [18].

Introductions of *M. bovis* into countries free of the organism have recently been reported (Finland 2012 [19], New Zealand 2017, (https://www.mpi.govt.nz/protection-and-response/mycoplasma-bovis/). Although these introductions have not been directly linked to semen, *M. bovis* risk, due to global semen trade, continues to be a concern, especially in New Zealand where eradication of *M. bovis* has been attempted. In this study, we evaluated the efficacy of the low OIE Code and the high CSS guideline GTLS concentrations and two ofloxacin concentrations on the viability of two different *M. bovis* strains in spiked frozen semen. We used an ATCC strain, as well as a wild type strain recently isolated from commercial AI semen straws [5]. Unlike in previous GTLS efficacy studies [10,12,13], we used a commercial animal protein free extender. We wanted to study if it was possible to achieve mycoplasmacidal effect, in other words, no detection of *M. bovis* in AI semen straws after semen was enriched in mycoplasma broth, and an aliquot of the broth culture was directly analyzed using *M. bovis* real-time polymerase chain reaction (PCR).

Mycoplasmas are fastidious organisms needing special culture media and expertise in isolation. Instead of mycoplasma culture, PCR could be an option in AI centers to ensure *M. bovis*-free semen lots. There are only a few studies about PCR detection of *M. bovis* in bovine semen. Therefore, we also evaluated sensitivity of different DNA extraction methods to detect *M. bovis* in semen.

Experiments to produce *M. bovis* contaminated AI straws were conducted, in a commercial AI straw producing laboratory, using industrial scale procedures. This was possible because semen production ceased in this center after these experiments.

2. Results

Raw pooled semen showed no growth in mycoplasma culture. *M. bovis* or Friis broth did not have any detrimental effect on quality parameters of semen (Table 1).

After storage of the AI straws for five weeks in liquid nitrogen, at high spiking concentrations (10^6 CFU/mL), viable *M. bovis* bacteria were detected in processed semen regardless of the processing protocol. When low *M. bovis* concentrations were inoculated, differences among processing protocols were seen (Table 2). At a low spiking concentration, the ATCC strain was more resistant than the wild type strain to different antibiotics. The only protocol inhibiting the growth of the ATCC strain was the high GTLS 500/100/300/600 μg/mL (final concentration in extended semen) supplement added in the semen lab to the extender. All protocols, except EU GTLS 250/50/150/300 μg/mL (final concentration in extended semen) and extender without antibiotics, inhibited the growth of the wild type at a low spiking concentration.

Table 1. Semen quality parameters of raw and spiked semen.

Semen	Strain (CFU/mL)	Motility %	Viability %	Sperm Concentration (10^6/mL)
Raw semen		75.0	82.5	1850
Processed semen	ATCC 10^3	55 ± 2.9	53 ± 3.0	65 ± 2.9
	ATCC 10^6	56 ± 6.1	53 ± 2.5	67 ± 2.3
	wild type 10^3	52 ± 5.5	52 ± 2.1	67 ± 2.1
	wild type 10^6	57 ± 5.5	52 ± 4.6	67 ± 2.3
	unspiked	53 ± 5.1	54 ± 2.3	61 ± 1.3

Table 2. Detection of *M. bovis* wild type and ATCC 27368 by culture (+/-) from three parallel pooled samples (e.g., + + +) from different antibiotic/extender protocols after five-week storage of the straws in liquid nitrogen. Concentration used in spiking and culture dilution are shown in the table.

	10^3 CFU/mL			10^6 CFU/mL		
Culture dilution	−2	−3	−4	−2	−3	−4
Wild type strain						
GTLS 500/100/300/600 [a]	- - -	- - -	- - -	- - -	+ + +	+ + +
CSS GTLS [b]	- - -	- - -	- - -	- - -	- - -	+ + +
EU GTLS [c]	- - -	- - +	- - -	- - -	+ + +	+ + +
OF 400 μg [d]	- - -	- - -	- - -	- - -	+ + +	+ + +
OF 100 μg	- - -	- - -	- - -	- - -	+ + +	+ + +
no antibiotic	+ + +	+ - +	+ - -	+ + +	+ + +	+ + +
ATCC strain						
GTLS 500/100/300/600	- - -	- - -	- - -	+ - -	- - -	+ + +
CSS GTLS	- - -	- - -	- + -	+ + +	- + -	+ + +
EU GTLS	- - -	+ + +	+ - -	- - -	+ + +	+ + +
OF 400 μg	- - -	- - +	+ - +	+ - +	+ + +	+ + +
OF 100 μg	- - -	+ + +	- + +	+ - -	+ + +	+ + +
no antibiotic	+ + +	+ + +	+ + -	+ + +	+ + +	+ + +

[a] gentamycin (500 μg/mL), tylosin (100 μg/mL), lincomycin (300 μg/mL), spectinomycin (600 μg/mL); [b] Certified Semen Services gentamycin (500 μg/mL), tylosin (100 μg/mL), lincomycin (300 μg/mL), spectinomycin (600 μg/mL) protocol; [c] gentamycin (250 μg/mL), tylosin (50 μg/mL), lincomycin (150 μg/mL), spectinomycin (300 μg/mL); [d] ofloxacin.

Antimicrobials present in extended semen affect the mycoplasma culture, and thus several dilutions were made. In samples with high concentration of antimicrobials, viable *M. bovis* could be detected only in the highest culture dilution (Table 2).

We compared three different DNA extraction methods for spiked semen samples. At a high spiking concentration (10^6 CFU/mL), all pools were positive in PCR regardless of the DNA extraction method. Ct values varied between 24.7 and 28.5, and no significant differences in Ct values among extraction methods were seen (data not shown).

At a low spiking concentration, the method using InstaGene™ (method three) was the most effective. Using this method, we detected *M. bovis* in 94% (17/18) of pools spiked with 10^3 CFU/mL of ATCC strain, and in 72% (13/18) spiked with 10^3 CFU/mL of wild type strain. With method one, 67% (12/18) and with method two, 56% (10/18) of pools spiked with ATCC strain were positive in PCR, respectively. For the wild type strain, respective figures were for method one 61% (11/18) and 33% (6/18) for method two (Table 3). The Ct values varied between 34.3 and 36.7, and no significant differences in Ct values among extraction methods were seen (data not shown).

Table 3. Comparison of three different DNA extraction methods for detection of *M. bovis* in semen using *oppD* real-time PCR. Results (+/-) from three parallel pools (e.g., + + +) from each antibiotic protocol are shown.

	10^3 CFU/mL						10^6 CFU/mL					
	ATCC			Wild Type			ATCC			Wild Type		
	Method 1 [a]	Method 2 [b]	Method 3 [c]	Method 1	Method 2	Method 3	Method 1	Method 2	Method 3	Method 1	Method 2	Method 3
GTLS 500/100/300/600	- + +	+ + -	+ + +	+ - -	+ - +	+ - -	+ + +	+ + +	+ + +	+ + +	+ + +	+ + +
CSS GTLS	+ - -	- + +	+ + +	- + +	- - -	+ + +	+ + +	+ + +	+ + +	+ + +	+ + +	+ + +
EU GTLS	+ + +	+ + -	+ + +	+ + +	+ - +	- + +	+ + +	+ + +	+ + +	+ + +	+ + +	+ + +
OF 400 µg	+ + +	+ - +	+ + +	+ - +	- - -	+ + -	+ + +	+ + +	+ + +	+ + +	+ + +	+ + +
OF 100 µg	- + -	- - +	+ - +	- + -	- - -	+ + +	+ + +	+ + +	+ + +	+ + +	+ + +	+ + +
Control	- + +	- - +	+ + +	- + +	+ + -	+ - +	+ + +	+ + +	+ + +	+ + +	+ + +	+ + +

[a] QIAamp DNA mini kit (Qiagen, Hilden, Germany); [b] 2% Triton-X 100 and QIAamp DNA mini kit (Parker et al. 2017); [c] InstaGene™ matrix (Bio-Rad, Helsinki, Finland).

Minimum inhibitory concentration values of the strains used in spiking are shown in Table 4.

Table 4. MIC values (µg/mL) of ATCC 27368 and wild type strains (dilution range of antibiotic tested).

Antibiotic	Dilution Range Tested µg/mL	ATCC 27368	Wild Type
Tylosin	0.5–32	≤0.5	16
Lincomycin	0.25–32	2	1
Spectinomycin	2–128	4	≤2
Enrofloxacin	0.03–2	0.25	0.25
Danofloxacin	0.03–2	0.25	0.25

3. Discussion

Our study showed that it is challenging to rely on the use of antibiotics in bovine semen production to control *M. bovis*. None of the studied antibiotics had any effect on viability of *M. bovis* at 10^6 CFU/mL in extended semen, and the lower spiking concentration of 10^3 CFU/mL gave discrepant results. The high GTLS concentration reduced the number of viable *M. bovis* below the level of detection in all but one pool when 10^3 CFU/mL was spiked. In contrast, using the low concentration EU GTLS protocol, four out of six pools were positive in culture, suggesting that the GTLS concentration stated in the OIE Code is not high enough to eliminate even a low concentration of *M. bovis* in semen.

Our results on efficacy of GTLS are in line with previous studies by Shin et al. [10] and Visser et al. [12,13], although there are marked differences in experimental setup among the studies. In our study, an AI straw production system was performed in a commercial facility using industrial scale procedures, the wild type study strain had been recently isolated from AI straws, different extenders and treatments were used, and survival of *M. bovis* was measured using a different method. In the earlier studies [10,12,13], animal protein containing extenders were used, as well as a plate counting method was used to detect viable *M. bovis*. Shin et al. [10] found that a high GTLS concentration in 20% egg yolk citrate extender showed 85% reduction of viable *M. bovis*. GTLS in other extenders was less mycoplasmacidal, thus, extender composition seemed to affect the efficacy of GTLS on *M. bovis*. However, the opinion of Shin et al. [10] was that the reduction of *M. bovis* concentration was so notable that it made the semen safe to use, and Shin's GTLS protocol was implemented for use in the Unites States AI industry. Later, Visser et al. [12,13] studied the effect of high GTLS in egg yolk tris extender. They noticed a one to two decimal reduction in *M. bovis* numbers in some batches, and in some batches the number of viable *M. bovis* was even higher in the GTLS-treated semen as compared with non-treated semen. We did not attempt to analyze the number of colony-forming units after liquid nitrogen storage. Instead, we aimed to find any viable *M. bovis* cells by enrichment culture and using real-time PCR to detect *M. bovis* in broth cultures. Previously, we showed that the limit of detection of this method was 1.4×10^2 CFU/mL of *M. bovis* PG45 in fresh, non-frozen extended bull semen [20]. Animal protein-free extender used in this study did not seem to enhance the efficacy of antibiotics as compared with earlier studies. The inclusion of further field strains isolated from AI semen in this study would have been appropriate, but these were not readily available.

Macrolide and linco/spectinomycin resistance, in recent *M. bovis* isolates from Europe, has increased as compared with isolates before 2000 [15,17]. This may have an impact on the effect of GTLS in *M. bovis* in semen as the highest dilutions tested in recent European studies [16,21] were from 64 to 256 µg/mL, and several strains had MIC values higher than the highest tested concentration. Antimicrobial susceptibility studies [15–17,21,22] showed that contemporary *M. bovis* strains are susceptible to fluoroquinolones, except for a few strains that had MIC_{90} over 32 µg/mL. Gloria et al. [18] reported that ofloxacin, a fluoroquinolone antibiotic, had non-significant effects on sperm quality and controlled bacteria efficiently in semen doses, although they did not study the effect on mycoplasmas. This tempted us to examine the effect of two different ofloxacin concentrations on *M. bovis* in semen. To our knowledge, this is the first publication on efficacy of a fluoroquinolone on *M. bovis* in commercial semen production. Although the ATCC strain used for spiking had an MIC value of 0.25 µg/mL for enrofloxacin and danofloxacin, the 100 µg/mL ofloxacin concentration in extender had no effect on the viability of the ATCC strain, and two out of three tested pools of the high ofloxacin concentration were also culture positive. Antimicrobial resistance, in the strains we used in this study did not explain the results, as MIC values for tylosin, lincomycin, and spectinomycin, as well as for fluoroquinolones, were well below the concentrations of antibiotics in semen extenders. The biological conditions for antibiotics to act with *M. bovis* in MIC testing are remarkably different as compared with conditions in semen production.

Most antibiotics require ongoing cell activity or cell division to be able to destroy bacteria. Low temperature can keep bacteria in a stationary phase of growth, thus, making the antibiotics almost ineffective. This is considered in the EU directive 88/407/1993 which states that extended semen with antibiotics must be kept a minimum of 45 min at 5 °C, and in the CSS protocol that requires, first, adding antibiotics in raw semen, and then keeping extended semen at 5 °C for a minimum of two hours before freezing. In our study, extended semen with different antibiotics was kept for 3–3.5 h at temperatures (decreasing from 34 °C to 17 °C) that, in theory, allowed replication of mycoplasmas. Thus, the negative effect of low temperature on antimicrobial effect cannot explain our results.

A possible way to control the dissemination of *M. bovis* via AI could be testing of raw semen or multiple straws of extended semen using PCR. However, PCR inhibitors present in semen can pose problems for detecting *M. bovis*. Semen contains very high amounts of DNA and protein, potassium ions, citric acids, and fructose. Therefore, it is essential to have a highly sensitive method for DNA isolation from bull semen. We compared three different DNA extraction methods and found that InstaGene™ proved to be the most efficient and robust method to detect *M. bovis* DNA in extended bull semen. To our knowledge, Parker et al. [23] and McDonald [24] are the only studies on the sensitivity of real-time PCR detection of *M. bovis* in semen. Parker et al. [23] used the Triton-X extraction method which, in our study, had lower sensitivity than the InstaGene™ method. Together with the *uvrC* gene-based real-time PCR, their limit of detection was 1.3×10^5 CFU/mL, which was higher than for our method. McDonald [24] used a commercial DNA isolation kit on spiked semen and multiplex real-time PCR targeting *fusA* and *oppD/F* genes. These assays detected 3.1×10^3 *M. bovis* genomes per mL semen, which was a similar level of detection to our InstaGene™ method. Little is known about shedding of *M. bovis* into semen during different stages of infection. It is generally known that shedding of mycoplasmas into semen can be intermittent. Ball et al. [25] showed that at least three semen lots from a bull needed to be analyzed to find out if the bull was shedding mycoplasmas into semen. This has also been shown for the secretion of *M. bovis* to semen. A clinically healthy bull in the AI center was shown to shed *M. bovis* in semen for a very short period and intermittently [5]. Our culture and PCR results also highlight the problem that *M. bovis* seems to be unequally distributed in extended semen, a phenomenon we also saw when examining the straws from the naturally infected bull semen. Therefore, it is important to analyze several straws, even from the same lot, when trying to detect *M. bovis* in semen. We also found that, within the same lot, some straws were positive only in PCR, but unculturable [5]. This can lead to unnecessary disposing of semen lots that contain only dead bacteria.

AI using *M. bovis*-contaminated semen can introduce the agent into naïve dairy herds. We showed that even using modern commercial extender and industrial procedures, neither GTLS nor ofloxacin reached 100% bactericidal effect on *M. bovis*. Our results suggest that regarding *M. bovis* in semen, it is safer to use the high 500/100/300/600 µg/mL GTLS concentration. To be able to fully understand the risk of *M. bovis* contaminated semen in dairy herds and to know if it is even necessary to have zero tolerance for *M. bovis* in commercial semen, we need to know what is the *M. bovis* load that would initiate a pathological process in the female genital system.

Another option, although very laborious, is to test processed semen for the presence of *M. bovis*, considering the special features of *M. bovis* infection in bulls and occurrence in semen. However, the increasing antimicrobial resistance in contemporary *M. bovis* strains, the difficulties achieving 100% mycoplasmacidal effect using antibiotics in semen, and the pressure to reduce the amount of antibiotics used in semen industry calls for future attempts to allow only *M. bovis* negative bulls into semen production.

4. Materials and Methods

4.1. Semen Collection and Quality Assessment

All studies were done in a commercial AI straw producing AI center's laboratory using industrial scale procedures. This was possible because the semen production ceased in this center after these experiments. Semen from three bulls was collected into sterile collection tubes at the AI center of VikingGenetics, Hollola, Finland. The motility of each semen batch was evaluated microscopically at 200× magnification using prewarmed glass slides and coverslips. Viability and concentration of each batch was analyzed using flow cytometry (CyFlow, Partec, Germany). Pooled raw semen (0.3 mL) was cultured in Friis broth [26] to detect possible *Mycoplasma* contamination. The final sperm cell concentration was 12–13 million per straw. On the basis of the weight and concentration, the volume of extender was calculated.

4.2. Mycoplasma Bovis Strains

Two *M. bovis* strains were used in spiking, i.e., a wild type isolate from commercial AI straws (strain 198, [5]) and a reference strain ATCC 27368. Strains were cultured in Friis broth in closed tubes at 37 °C, for 70 ± 2 h. High (10^8 CFU/mL) and low (10^5 CFU/mL) concentration stock solutions were made from the cultures in Friis broth. To verify the *M. bovis* concentration of the stocks, ten-fold dilutions were made and plated on Friis plates. Plates were incubated at 37 °C, in 5% CO_2, for 7 days, and colony-forming units were counted.

4.3. Protocols Used for Processing Semen

Semen from the three bulls was pooled and divided into 30 aliquots which were kept at 32 °C. Commercial animal protein-free extender base containing 7% glycerol was used in all protocols. Six antibiotic protocols were compared as follows: (1) GTLS (500/100/300/600 μg/mL, respectively) fresh antibiotic supplemented extender; (2) raw semen was treated with GTLS fresh antibiotics for 3 min and further extended with GTLS (500/100/300/600 μg/mL, respectively) fresh antibiotic supplemented extender (according to Certified Semen Services (CSS) requirements), later called CSS GTLS; (3) GTLS (250/50/150/300 μg/mL, respectively), antibiotic supplemented extender (ready to use liquid concentrate containing antibiotics), according to the OIE Code, Article 4.7.7, later called EU GTLS; (4) ofloxacin 100 μg/mL (Sigma Aldrich 33703) antibiotic supplemented extender; or (5) ofloxacin 400 μg/mL antibiotic supplemented extender; and (6) extender without antibiotics, control. The final concentration of the *M. bovis* strains in extended semen was either 10^6 CFU/mL or 10^3 CFU/mL. Friis broth was used as a negative control in each different antibiotic/extender aliquot. The protocols are described in Table 5. All extenders, antibiotics, and Friis broth were kept at 32 °C before being added into the semen. All protocols, except number two (CSS GTLS), included diluting the semen in 1:1extender (with or without antibiotics) and Friis broth containing either 10^8 or 10^5 CFU *M. bovis* ATCC or wild type. In protocol two (CSS GTLS), GTLS was first diluted 1:4 in sterile water and 38 μL added into neat semen (380 μL), *M. bovis* culture (118 μL) yielding the same antibiotic concentration as if 20 μL GTLS mixture (500/100/300/600) would have been added directly to raw semen. After 3 min of incubation at 32 °C, the semen was further diluted 1:1 with extender containing GTLS. Then, all aliquots were incubated for one hour at 34 °C, after which they were diluted further with extender with or without antibiotics to give the final concentration of 56 million sperm cells/mL. Then, the temperature of the aliquots was allowed to stabilize to room temperature (approximately one hour) after which automatic semen straw filling and sealing machine (MPP Quattro, Minitube, Germany) was used. Semen was packed into 0.25 mL straws. After packing, the straws were cooled to 17 °C for one hour and further cooled quickly to 4 °C. The straws were kept at 4 °C overnight and they were deep-frozen with industrial semen straw freezer (Digitcool 5300, IMV, France) the next morning. Cryopreserved straws were stored in liquid nitrogen storage tank (−196 °C) until they were analyzed.

Table 5. Antibiotic/extender protocols used for processing semen.

GTLS (500/100/300/600)	CSS GTLS (500/100/300/600)	EU GTLS (250/50/150/300)	OF400	OF100	Control
0.38 mL semen	0.38 mL semen	0.38 mL semen	0.38 mL semen	0.38 mL semen	0.38 mL semen
+	+	+	+	+	+
0.38 mL GTLS extender	0.118 mL *M.bovis*	0.38 mL GTLS extender	0.38 mL OF extender	0.38 mL OF extender	0.38 mL extender no antibiotic
+	+	+	+	+	+
0.118 mL *M. bovis*	38 µL GTLS 1:4 3 min	0.118 mL *M. bovis*	0.118 mL *M. bovis*	0.118 mL *M. bovis*	0.118 mL *M. bovis*
+	+	+	+	+	+
	0.38 mL GTLS extender				
	+				
1 h 34 °C	1 h 34 °C	1 h 34 °C	1 h 34 °C	1 h 34 °C	1 h 34 °C
+	+	+	+	+	+
10.875 mL GTLS extender	10.875 mL GTLS extender	10.875 mL GTLS extender	10.875 mL OF extender	10.875 mL OF extender	10.875 mL extender no antibiotic
Room temperature 50–90 min and packing in straws (0.25 mL per straw) 1 h + 17 °C 21 h + 4 °C Storage in liquid nitrogen					

4.4. Semen Quality Parameters after Thawing

After 18 days storage in liquid nitrogen, two straws from each trial lot were thawed. The motility was assessed under phase contrast microscope. Flow cytometric analysis was used to evaluate viability and concentration of sperm cells.

4.5. Viability Testing of M. Bovis from Semen Straws Stored in Liquid Nitrogen

After storage of five weeks in liquid nitrogen, 18 straws from each of the 30 trial lots were randomly retrieved from the nitrogen tank. They were divided into three pools, each consisting of six straws. Straws were thawed and the content of the six straws was pooled. From each pool, 0.6 mL of semen was used in three different DNA extraction procedures described in Section 4.6., and 0.3 mL of semen was placed into 2.7 mL of Friis broth. Ten-fold dilutions, up to 10^{-5}, were made into Friis broth in tightly closed tubes. Broth cultures were incubated at 37 °C for 14 days. The growth and color change of the medium were monitored every other day, and broths suspected of mycoplasma growth were plated on Friis agar and tested for *M. bovis* using real-time PCR targeting *M. bovis oppD* gene [27]. From each trial lot, all broth culture dilutions from 10^{-2} to 10^{-4} were tested for *M. bovis*, as described above, at the latest, immediately after the 14-day incubation period.

4.6. DNA Extraction from Semen Straws after Storage in Liquid Nitrogen

Three different protocols to extract DNA from spiked semen were compared. In each method, 200 µL of semen was used as a starting material. Method one was automated DNA extraction using a QIAcube (Qiagen, Hilden, Germany) robot and blood and body fluids protocol with QIAamp DNA mini kit. The elution volume was 150 µL. In method two [25], 200 µL of semen was combined with 200 µL of 2% Triton-X 100 (Sigma Aldrich) in 10 mM Tris and 1 mM EDTA (pH 8) buffer. The sample was thoroughly vortexed and pelleted at 13,000× *g* for 5 min. DNA was extracted from the pellet using the QIAcube robot and bacterial pellet protocol with QIAamp DNA mini kit. The elution volume was 150 µL. Method three was modified from the OIE Terrestrial Manual method to isolate DNA from bovine semen for herpesvirus PCR (chapter 3.4.11, adopted May 2017). In method three, 200 µL of semen was centrifuged at 13,000× *g* for 10 min and supernatant was discarded. The pellet was mixed with 200 µL of InstaGene™ matrix (Bio-Rad, Helsinki, Finland), 5.8 µL proteinase K (20 mg/mL), and 7.5 µL DL-dithiothreitol (1 M). Samples were incubated at 56 °C, for 30 min, and then vortexed at high speed for 10 s. The tubes were boiled in water bath (100 °C) for 8 min, and then vortexed at high speed for 10 s. Then, the tubes were centrifuged at 10,000× *g* for 3 min. The supernatant was transferred into a new microtube and stored at −20 °C.

4.7. M. bovis Real-Time PCR

Broth cultures and DNA extracted from semen straw pools were examined by real-time PCR (CFX96 Touch Real-Time PCR Detection System, Bio-Rad, CA, USA) targeting *opp*D-gene of *M. bovis*, as described previously by Sachse et al [27]. Friis broth cultures were prepared for real-time PCR as follows: First, 200 µL of broth culture was incubated for 15 min at 95 °C and centrifuged at 10,000× *g* for 5 min. Two µL of culture supernatant or DNA was used as PCR template. Commercially available plasmid pUC19 was used as internal amplification control, according to Fricker et al. [28].

4.8. Determining Minimal Inhibitory Concentration (MIC) of Wild Type Strain and ATCC 27368

MICs were determined using custom made Sensititre plates (Thermo Fisher Scientific, UK). Antibiotics tested were tylosin (concentration range 0.5–32 µg/mL), lincomycin (0.25–32 µg/mL), spectinomycin (2–128 µg/mL), enrofloxacin (0.03–2 µg/mL), and danofloxacin (0.03–2 µg/mL). Testing was done according to [15,16]. Briefly, a suspension containing 5% growth indicator alamarBlue (Thermo Fisher Scientific, United Kingdom) in Friis broth without antibiotics and *M. bovis* 5×10^5 CFU/mL was made, and 200 µL of the suspension was pipetted into each well of the Sensititre plate. Plates were sealed and incubated at 37 °C for 48 ± 1 h and read visually; blue indicating no growth and red indicating growth of the isolate. MIC was the lowest concentration of antibiotic completely suppressing growth (blue color).

Author Contributions: Conceptualization, T.P., N.V., T.A., and S.P.; methodology, T.P., N.V., and T.A.; formal analysis, T.P., N.V., and T.A.; investigation, N.V. and H.S.; resources, H.S.; writing—original draft preparation, T.P.; writing—review and editing, T.P., T.A., H.S., and S.P.; supervision, T.A.; project administration and funding acquisition, S.P. All authors have read and agreed to the published version of the manuscript.

Funding: This research was funded by the Ministry of Agriculture and Forestry of Finland, grant number 1490/03.01.02//2016.

Acknowledgments: We are grateful to Riikka Luukkanen and Petra Väisänen for excellent technical assistance. We thank DVM Kasia Kupisiewicz for critical reding of the manuscript.

Conflicts of Interest: Henri Simonen is employed by VikingGenetics, however, experiments, interpretation of results, and manuscript preparation has been done independently. The funders had no role in the design of the study; in the collection, analyses, or interpretation of data; in the writing of the manuscript, or in the decision to publish the results.

References

1. Maunsell, F.P.; Woolums, A.R.; Francoz, D.; Rosenbusch, R.F.; Step, D.L.; Wilson, D.J.; Janzen, E.D. Mycoplasma bovis infections in cattle. *J. Vet. Intern. Med.* **2011**, *25*, 772–783. [CrossRef] [PubMed]
2. Perez-Casal, J.; Prysliak, T.; Maina, T.; Suleman, M.; Jimbo, S. Status of the development of a vaccine against Mycoplasma bovis. *Vaccine* **2017**, *35*, 2902–2907. [CrossRef] [PubMed]
3. Nicholas, R.A. Bovine mycoplasmosis: Silent and deadly. *Vet. Rec.* **2011**, *168*, 459–462. [CrossRef]
4. Pfützner, H.; Sachse, K. Mycoplasma bovis as an agent of mastitis, pneumonia, arthritis and genital disorders in cattle. *Rev. Sci. Tech.* **1996**, *15*, 1477–1494. [CrossRef]
5. Haapala, V.; Pohjanvirta, T.; Vähänikkilä, N.; Halkilahti, J.; Simonen, H.; Pelkonen, S.; Soveri, T.; Simojoki, H.; Autio, T. Semen as a source of Mycoplasma bovis mastitis in dairy herds. *Vet. Microbiol.* **2018**, *216*, 60–66. [CrossRef] [PubMed]
6. Hirth, R.S.; Nielsen, S.W.; Plastridge, W.N. Bovine salpingo-oophoritis produced with semen containing a Mycoplasma. *Pathol. Vet.* **1966**, *3*, 616–632. [CrossRef]
7. Kissi, B.; Juhász, S.; Stipkovits, L. Effect of mycoplasma contamination of bull semen on fertilization. *Acta Vet. Hung.* **1985**, *33*, 107–117.
8. Wentink, G.H.; Frankena, K.; Bosch, J.C.; Vandehoek, J.E.D.; van den Berg, T. Prevention of disease transmission by semen in cattle. *Livest. Prod. Sci.* **2000**, *62*, 207–220. [CrossRef]
9. OIE Terrestrial Animal Health Code, Chapter 4.7. Available online: https://www.oie.int/index.php?id=169&L=0&htmfile=chapitre_coll_semen.htm (accessed on 5 August 2020).
10. Shin, S.J.; Lein, D.H.; Patten, V.H.; Ruhnke, H.L. A new antibiotic combination for frozen bovine semen 1. Control of mycoplasmas, ureaplasmas, Campylobacter fetus subsp. venerealis and Haemophilus somnus. *Theriogenology* **1988**, *29*, 577–591. [CrossRef]
11. CSS—National Association of Animal Breeders. Available online: https://www.naab-css.org/uploads/userfiles/files/CSSMinReq-Jan2014201607-ENG.pdf (accessed on 5 August 2020).
12. Visser, I.J.R.; ter Laak, E.A.; Jansen, H.B.; Gerard, O. The effect of antibiotic mixtures on Haemophilus somnus, Campylobacter fetus spp. venerealis, Mycoplasma bovis, and Ureaplasma diversum in frozen bovine semen. *Reprod. Domest. Anim.* **1995**, *30*, 55–59. [CrossRef]
13. Visser, I.J.; ter Laak, E.A.; Jansen, H.B. Failure of antibiotics gentamycin, tylosin, lincomycin and spectinomycin to eliminate Mycoplasma bovis in artificially infected frozen bovine semen. *Theriogenology* **1999**, *51*, 689–697. [CrossRef]
14. Rehman, F.; Zhao, C.; Shah, M.A.; Qureshi, M.S.; Wang, X. Semen extenders and artificial insemination in ruminants. *Veterinaria* **2013**, *1*, 1–8.
15. Ayling, R.D.; Rosales, R.S.; Barden, G.; Gosney, F.L. Changes in antimicrobial susceptibility of Mycoplasma bovis isolates from Great Britain. *Vet. Rec.* **2014**, *175*, 486. [CrossRef] [PubMed]
16. Heuvelink, A.; Reugebrink, C.; Mars, J. Antimicrobial susceptibility of Mycoplasma bovis isolates from veal calves and dairy cattle in the Netherlands. *Vet. Microbiol.* **2016**, *189*, 1–7. [CrossRef]

17. Klein, U.; de Jong, A.; Youala, M.; El Garch, F.; Stevenin, C.; Moyaert, H.; Rose, M.; Catania, S.; Gyuranecz, M.; Pridmore, A.; et al. New antimicrobial susceptibility data from monitoring of Mycoplasma bovis isolated in Europe. *Vet. Microbiol.* **2019**, *238*, 108432. [CrossRef]
18. Gloria, A.; Contri, A.; Wegher, L.; Vignola, G.; Dellamaria, D.; Carluccio, A. The effects of antibiotic additions to extenders on fresh and frozen-thawed bull semen. *Anim. Reprod. Sci.* **2014**, *150*, 15–23. [CrossRef] [PubMed]
19. Vähänikkilä, N.; Pohjanvirta, T.; Haapala, V.; Simojoki, H.; Soveri, T.; Browning, G.F.; Pelkonen, S.; Wawegama, N.K.; Autio, T. Characterisation of the course of Mycoplasma bovis infection in naturally infected dairy herds. *Vet. Microbiol.* **2019**, *231*, 107–115. [CrossRef]
20. Vähänikkilä, N.; Pohjanvirta, T.; Vaahtoranta, L.; Silvennoinen, M.; Skovgaard Jensen, S.K.; Pelkonen, S.; Autio, T. Detection of Mycoplasma bovis in bovine semen—An interlaboratory trial. In Proceedings of the 22nd Congress of the International Organization for Mycoplasmology, Portsmouth, NH, USA, 9–12 July 2018; Brown, D., Wells, N., Eds.; p. 143.
21. Sulyok, K.M.; Kreizinger, Z.; Fekete, L.; Hrivnák, V.; Magyar, T.; Jánosi, S.; Schweitzer, N.; Turcsányi, I.; Makrai, L.; Erdélyi, K.; et al. Antibiotic susceptibility profiles of Mycoplasma bovis strains isolated from cattle in Hungary, Central Europe. *BMC Vet. Res.* **2014**, *10*, 256. [CrossRef]
22. Gautier-Bouchardon, A.V.; Ferré, S.; Le Grand, D.; Paoli, A.; Gay, E.; Poumarat, F. Overall decrease in the susceptibility of Mycoplasma bovis to antimicrobials over the past 30 years in France. *PLoS ONE* **2014**, *9*, e87672. [CrossRef]
23. Parker, A.M.; House, J.K.; Hazelton, M.S.; Bosward, K.L.; Sheehy, P.A. Comparison of culture and a multiplex probe PCR for identifying Mycoplasma species in bovine milk, semen and swab samples. *PLoS ONE* **2017**, *12*, e0173422. [CrossRef]
24. McDonald, K.M. The Development of a Dual Target Mycoplasma Bovis TaqMan Real-Time PCR System for Rapid Analysis of Bovine Semen. Master's Thesis, The Ohio State University, Columbus, OH, USA, 2012.
25. Ball, H.J.; Logan, E.F.; Orr, W. Isolation of mycoplasmas from bovine semen in Northern Ireland. *Vet. Rec.* **1987**, *121*, 322–324. [CrossRef] [PubMed]
26. Bölske, G. Survey of mycoplasma infections in cell cultures and a comparison of detection methods. *Zentralbl. Bakteriol. Mikrobiol. Hyg. Ser. A* **1988**, *269*, 331–340. [CrossRef]
27. Sachse, K.; Salam, H.S.H.; Diller, R.; Schubert, E.; Hoffmann, B.; Hotzel, H. Use of a novel real-time PCR technique to monitor and quantitate Mycoplasma bovis infection in cattle herds with mastitis and respiratory disease. *Vet. J.* **2010**, *186*, 299–303. [CrossRef] [PubMed]
28. Fricker, M.; Messelhäußer, U.; Busch, U.; Schere, S.; Ehling-Schultz, M. Diagnostic real-time PCR assays fot the detection of emetic Bacillus cereus strains in food and recent food-borne outbreaks. *Appl. Environ. Microbiol.* **2007**, *73*, 1892–1898. [CrossRef] [PubMed]

pathogens

MDPI

Article

Identification of Antimicrobial Resistance-Associated Genes through Whole Genome Sequencing of *Mycoplasma bovis* Isolates with Different Antimicrobial Resistances

Lisa Ledger, Jason Eidt and Hugh Y. Cai *

Animal Health Lab, University of Guelph, 419 Gordon St., Guelph, ON N1H 6R8, Canada; lledger@uoguelph.ca (L.L.); jeidt@uoguelph.ca (J.E.)

* Correspondence: hcai@uoguelph.ca

Received: 30 June 2020; Accepted: 16 July 2020; Published: 19 July 2020

Abstract: Antimicrobial resistance (AMR) in *Mycoplasma bovis* has been previously associated with topoisomerase and ribosomal gene mutations rather than specific resistance-conferring genes. Using whole genome sequencing (WGS) to identify potential new AMR mechanisms for *M. bovis*, it was found that a 2019 clinical isolate with high MIC (2019-043682) for fluoroquinolones, macrolides, lincosamides, pleuromutilins and tetracyclines had a new core genome multilocus sequencing (cgMLST) type (ST10-like) and 91% sequence similarity to the published genome of *M. bovis* PG45. Closely related to PG45, a 1982 isolate (1982-M6152) shared the same cgMLST type (ST17), 97.2% sequence similarity and low MIC results. Known and potential AMR- associated genetic events were identified through multiple sequence alignment of the three genomes. Isolate 2019-043682 had 507 genes with non-synonymous mutations (NSMs) and 67 genes disrupted. Isolate 1982-M6152 had 81 NSMs and 20 disruptions. Using functional roles and known mechanisms of antimicrobials, a 55 gene subset was assessed for AMR potential. Seventeen were previously identified from other bacteria as sites of AMR mutation, 38 shared similar functions to them, and 11 contained gene-disrupting mutations. This study indicated that *M. bovis* may obtain high AMR characteristics by mutating or disrupting other functional genes, in addition to topoisomerases and ribosomal genes.

Keywords: *Mycoplasma bovis*; antimicrobial resistance; whole genome sequencing; MIC; cgMLST

---

1. Introduction

Mycoplasma bovis is a member of the Mollicutes; membrane-bound bacteria which lack a cell wall, precluding the use of many common antimicrobial agents such as the β-lactams [1]. In cattle, *M. bovis* is a causative agent of pneumonia, arthritis, otitis media, and reproductive disease and is a contributor to the bovine respiratory disease (BRD) complex, also known as 'shipping fever', which is a major source of morbidity, mortality and financial loss in calf and feedlot operations. Additionally, *M. bovis* is capable of persisting for the life of a colonized animal, which may remain asymptomatic while acting as a source of infection for herdmates or offspring [1,2].

Of note, many of the antibiotics to which *M. bovis* shows resistance are not licensed for usage in treating *M. bovis* infections [3] but may be used in the treatment of other bovine bacterial pathogens. Given the asymptomatic nature of many *M. bovis* infections, and the high rates of colonization when animals are co-mingled (potentially over 90%) [4,5], conditions are favourable for the development of multi-drug resistant strains. With global rates of antimicrobial resistance increasing, understanding the molecular mechanisms underlying antimicrobial resistance, particularly for multi-drug resistant (MDR) strains, is critical for determining effective treatment [6], or potentially to design treatment protocols that use evolutionary approaches to counter or reverse antimicrobial resistance [7].

Unlike other members of the BRD complex such as *Mannheimia haemolytica*, *Histophilus somni* or *Pasteurella multocida*, *M. bovis* is not known to possess defined antimicrobial resistance genes [8] but appears to have the molecular mechanisms of its resistance rooted in point mutations within several ribosomal and topoisomerase genes. Previous studies have used whole-genome sequencing (WGS) paired with minimum inhibitory concentration (MIC) testing to establish that mutations within *gyrA* and *parC* are linked to increased resistance to fluoroquinolones, that increased resistance to spectinomycin and the tetracyclines is linked to *rrs1-rrs2* (16S rRNA gene) mutations, and that *rrl1-rrl2* (23S rRNA gene) mutations are linked to increased resistance to florfenicol, lincosamides, macrolides and pleuromutilins [9], with *rrl3* (23S rRNA gene) also implicated in macrolide resistance [10].

In a large-scale MIC study of *M. bovis* strains isolated between 1978 to 2009, fluctuations in antimicrobial susceptibility over time were observed [3] with the MIC50 values, and thus resistance, increasing for several tetracycline and macrolide-class antimicrobial drugs over the span of the study. Additionally, associations between MIC50 values were observed for different antimicrobials; although sequencing these isolates fell beyond the scope of the study, the association between lincosamides, pleuromutilins and florfenicol in terms of *rrl1-rrl2* mutations was mirrored by a similar observed association in MIC50 values with these historical samples.

A high MIC *M. bovis* was isolated from lung tissues of a two-week old male Holstein calf submitted to the Animal Health Lab in July of 2019 for post-mortem examination. In the interest of determining possible genetic factors for this high level of resistance, whole-genome sequencing using the Illumina MiSeq platform was conducted, in tandem with WGS of a historical isolate of *M. bovis* (1982-M6152) previously categorized as low MIC for most antimicrobials [3]. The MICs and sequence data for both isolates were compared to *M. bovis* strain PG45, a reference strain with a fully sequenced and circularized genome, in order to identify any gaps in sequencing coverage, to determine if any new genes were present in the isolates as opposed to a reference strain, and to better elucidate which mutations in the high MIC isolate were potentially significant for AMR by ruling out any shared mutations with the low MIC isolate.

2. Results

2.1. MIC Testing

Cultures of two isolates of *M. bovis* (1982-M6152 and 2019-043682) and *M. bovis* strain PG45 (used as a reference strain) were tested in triplicate for minimum inhibitory concentration of 16 antimicrobials (Table 1), with the results of MIC testing identical within each triplicate. Relative to *M. bovis* PG45, isolate 1982-M6152 shows a two-fold increase in MIC for oxytetracycline but is otherwise identical in response to other antimicrobial compounds. Isolate 2019-043682 shows increased MICs for multiple fluoroquinolones, macrolides and tetracyclines, as well as a lincosamide, a pleuromutilin and two inhibitors of protein synthesis (gentamicin and florfenicol). For aminoglycosides the results are mixed, with increased MIC observed for spectinomycin, but no change in MIC for neomycin. All three strains have high MICs for sulfonamides, although they retain a low MIC for combination trimethoprim/sulfa.

2.2. Whole-Genome Sequencing

Raw sequencing yield for the two sequenced isolates was 167.8 Mb for 1982-M6152 (GenBank accession: CP058969), and 54.02 Mb for 2019-043682 (GenBank accession: CP058968). Given the sequencing yields and the documented genome size of 1.003 Mb for *M. bovis* PG45 (GenBank accession NC_014760.1), raw sequencing coverage (where C = yield/genome size) was 167× for 1982-M6152 and 54× for 2019-043682, which is sufficient for analysis of mutations and SNPs. Assembled using SPAdes 3.9.0 [11] in Illumina's BaseSpace hub (Illumina, Inc., San Diego, CA, USA) genome sizes were 978,895 bp for 1982-M6152 and 941,076 bp for 2019-043682. Also within BaseSpace, core genome multilocus squence typing (cgMLST) was conducted for both isolates sequenced, using Bacterial

Analysis Pipeline v1.0.4 [12]. Isolate 2019-043682 had an undescribed cgMLST type (ST10-like) while isolate 1982-M6152 had the same cgMLST type (ST17) as PG45.

Table 1. Average results of MIC testing for two isolates of Mycoplasma bovis, compared to reference strain PG45, by μg of antimicrobial compound required to inhibit growth. Isolates and the reference strain were tested in triplicate with identical results within each triplicate for all antimicrobials tested.

Antimicrobial	PG45	2019-043682	1982-M6152
Neomycin	>32	>32	>32
Spectinomycin	<8	16	<8
Trimethoprim/Sulfa	>2/38	>2/38	>2/38
Danofloxacin	0.5	>1	0.5
Enrofloxacin	0.5	2	0.5
Clindamycin	<0.25	>16	<0.25
Tilmicosin	<4	>64	<4
Tulathromycin	8	>64	8
Tylosin Tartrate	1	>32	1
Tiamulin	1	8	1
Gentamicin	8	16	8
Florfenicol	4	>8	4
Sulphadimethoxine	>256	>256	>256
Chlortetracycline	<0.5	>8	<0.5
Oxytetracycline	<0.5	>8	1
Ceftiofur	>8	>8	>8

Assembly and multiple sequence alignment (MSA) of both isolates with *M. bovis* PG45 in Geneious 11(Biomatters, Auckland, New Zealand) (Figure 1) revealed that 2019-043682 had 91% sequence similarity to PG45. 1982-M6152 had 97.2% sequence similarity to PG4.

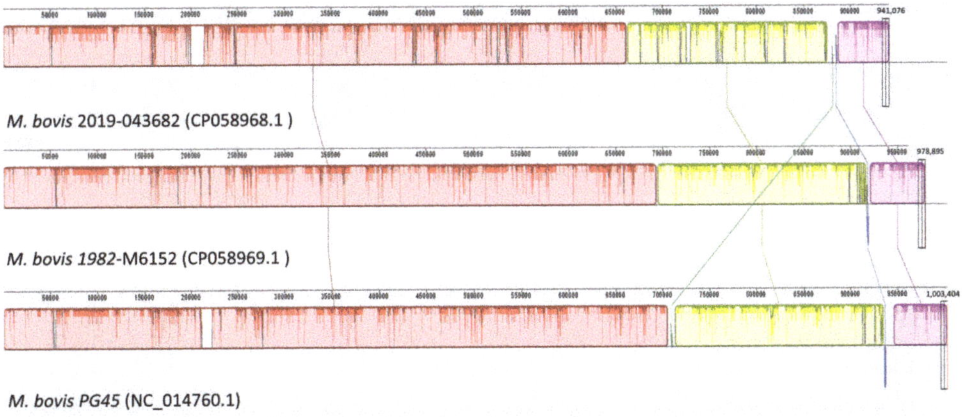

Figure 1. Graphical output of multiple sequence alignment (Mauve, Geneious 11) for *M. bovis* isolates 2019-43682, 1982-M6152 and *M. bvis* strain *PG45* with GenBank accessions displaying depth of sequencing and areas with large deletions.

Annotation of the MSA in MegAlign using feature data for PG45 identified 878 features (MegAlign's term: CDS, in more general usage) in strain PG45, with divergences by isolate summarized in Table 2. Features were reported as Identical by MegAlign if they were 100% identical to PG45, with 100% coverage. Features were reported as Not_Mapped by MegAlign if their % identity score fell below 95%. Unmapped features have been further categorized by the researchers as excised, truncated or highly variable based on their % coverage score (Table 2). Isolate 1982-M6152 had 696 features identical to PG45, 105 with substitutions, 37 with insertions or deletions and 39 reported as Not_Mapped.

Of these 39, 24 were excised, 11 truncated and 4 present but highly variable. Isolate 2019-043682 had 183 identical features, 471 with substitutions, 50 with insertions or deletions, and 173 reported as Not_Mapped. Of these, 81 were excised, 48 were truncated, and 44 were present but highly variable. Although several features were excised in the isolates relative to PG45, no unique features were identified in either isolate that were absent from PG45.

Table 2. Summary of variation of isolates from *M. bovis* PG45, by feature count (CDS), generated using MegAlign. v17 for multiple sequence alignment.

Genetic Events		1982-M6152	2019-043682
Variation types	Identical	696	183
	Deletion	8	18
	Deleted_end_3prime	3	3
	Deleted_end_5prime	1	3
	Indel	3	4
	Insertion	22	22
	Not_Mapped	39	173
	Substitution	105	471
	TOTAL	877	877
Unmapped features	Excised (<5% coverage)	24	81
	Truncated (5–95% coverage)	11	48
	Highly variable (>95% coverage)	4	44
	TOTAL	39	173

To determine which mutations could potentially alter gene function, further analysis of the two isolates using DNAStar's ArrayStar software revealed 3285 individual nonsynonymous mutations relative to *M. bovis* PG45 in total between the two isolates, across 513 genes and pseudogenes. Isolate 1982-M6152 contained 81 genes with non-synonymous mutations, 20 of which were disrupted. Isolate 2019-043682 contained 507 genes with non-synonymous mutations, with 67 genes disrupted. 17 genes with non-synonymous mutations were common to both isolate 1982-M6152 and isolate 2019-043682, with 14 of the mutations identical between the 2 isolates. Four genes with disrupting mutations were common to both isolates, with an insertion mutation in gene MBOVPG45_RS03940 (insertion TTGT, PG45 genome reference position 918372) identical between isolates. A subset of 55 genes (Table 3) containing NSMs was selected for further consideration based on the functional role of the genes and known mechanisms of antimicrobials, through consultation of the Comprehensive Antibiotic Resistance Database (CARD) and literature review [13]. Additionally, 22 genes were identified as ABC transporter system genes (Table 4) although the lack of available characterization has led to them being grouped separately for discussion. A full list of nonsynonymous mutations, their sequence and their positions is available as supplementary data (Supplementary Tables S1 and S2), as well as an expanded version of Table 3 (Supplementary Table S3) containing gene descriptions.

Table 3. Count of non-synonymous mutations (NSMs) relative to *M. bovis* PG45, by gene and by isolate, for a subset of NSM-containing genes identified as potentially associated with antimicrobial resistance.

Functional Role:	Gene:	1982-M6152	2019-043682	Associated AMR:	Reference:
Topoisomerases	gyrA	0	8	fluoroquinolones	[9]
	gyrB	0	6	fluoroquinolones	[9]
	parC	1 *	19 *	fluoroquinolones	[9]
	parE	0	4	fluoroquinolones	[14]
	topA	0	1 ^		

Table 3. *Cont.*

Functional Role:	Gene:	1982-M6152	2019-043682	Associated AMR:	Reference:
Protein Synthesis:					
Methyltransferases:	MBOVPG45_RS00465	0	2		
	MBOVPG45_RS00470	0	7		
	MBOVPG45_RS02280	0	4		
	rlmB	0	5	Predicted AMR	[15]
	rlmD	0	11		
	rlmH	0	1		
	rsmA	0	6	aminoglycosides	[16]
	rsmD	0	1	aminoglycosides	[16]
	rsmH	0	5	aminoglycosides	[16]
	rsmI	0	5	aminoglycosides	[16]
	trmB	0	4 ^		
30S Ribosomal Proteins	rpsB	0	3	aminoglycosides	[17]
	rpsC	2	1	tetracyclines	[18]
	rpsD	0	2		
	rpsE	1	2	aminoglycosides	[19]
	rpsH	0	1		
	rpsJ	1	0	tetracyclines	[20]
	rpsP	0	2		
	rpsS	0	1		
	rbfA	0	1		
50S Ribosomal Proteins	MBOVPG45_RS00445	0	1		
	rplB	0	1		
	rplC	0	1	pleuromutilins	[21]
	rplD	0	10	linezolid	[22]
	MBOVPG45_RS03525	0	2		
	rplV	0	1	macrolides	[23]
	MBOVPG45_RS01360	0	1		
	rpmE	0	1	MDR	[24]
tRNA ligases	alaS	1	8 ^	novobiocin	[25]
	MBOVPG45_RS01640	0	5		
	asnS	0	1	multi-drug resistance	[26]
	MBOVPG45_RS00205	0	9		
	MBOVPG45_RS01150	0	6 ^		
	MBOVPG45_RS02730	0	2		
	MBOVPG45_RS02640	0	1		
	ileS	1	5 ^	pseudomonic acid	[27]
	MBOVPG45_RS03145	0	1		
	MBOVPG45_RS02255	0	16		
	lysS	0	3	methicillin	[28]
	MBOVPG45_RS03150	0	10		
	pheS	0	2	MDR	[26]
	MBOVPG45_RS00380	0	18		
	serS	0	1		
tRNA ligases	MBOVPG45_RS02170	1	8 ^		
	trpS	0	1		
	MBOVPG45_RS04210	0	9 ^		
	MBOVPG45_RS00740	0	7 ^		
	tilS	0	8		
	thiI	0	4		
	mnmA	0	5		

* Identical NSM; ^ Contains a gene-disrupting NSM.

Table 4. Count of non-synonymous mutations (NSMs) relative to *M. bovis* PG45, by gene and by isolate, for ABC transporter system genes potentially linked to the bacterial efflux pump mechanism of AMR. ^Gene contains a disrupting mutation.

Gene:	1982-M6152	2019-043682	Description:
MBOVPG45_RS00090	0	1	ABC transporter ATP-binding protein
MBOVPG45_RS00180	0	2	ABC transporter permease
MBOVPG45_RS00555	0	2	ABC transporter permease
MBOVPG45_RS00570	0	4	ATP-binding cassette domain-containing protein
MBOVPG45_RS00600	0	1	ATP-binding cassette domain-containing protein
MBOVPG45_RS01485	0	2	energy-coupling factor transporter transmembrane protein EcfT
MBOVPG45_RS01540	0	1	sugar ABC transporter permease
MBOVPG45_RS01545	0	4	ATP-binding cassette domain-containing protein
MBOVPG45_RS01720	0	1	ABC transporter permease subunit
MBOVPG45_RS01770	0	1	ABC transporter ATP-binding protein
MBOVPG45_RS01775	1	7	ABC transporter permease
MBOVPG45_RS02005	0	5	ABC transporter ATP-binding protein
MBOVPG45_RS02710	0	1	ABC transporter permease subunit
MBOVPG45_RS02715	0	2	ATP-binding cassette domain-containing protein
MBOVPG45_RS02905	1	1	ABC transporter permease subunit
MBOVPG45_RS03425	0	1	ATP-binding cassette domain-containing protein
MBOVPG45_RS03465	0	4	ABC transporter ATP-binding protein
MBOVPG45_RS03470	0	6	ABC transporter ATP-binding protein
MBOVPG45_RS03705	0	6 ^	carbohydrate ABC transporter permease
MBOVPG45_RS03710	0	1	sugar ABC transporter permease
MBOVPG45_RS04310	0	5	ABC transporter ATP-binding protein
MBOVPG45_RS04315	1	89	ABC transporter permease

^ Contains a gene-disrupting NSM.

3. Discussion

The recent isolate 2019-043682 had significantly elevated MICs for multiple fluoroquinolones, macrolides and tetracyclines, as well as a lincosamide, a pleuromutilin, spectinomycin, and two inhibitors of protein synthesis (gentamicin and florfenicol), indicating multi-drug resistant *M. bovis* can emerge in the field.

Of the *M. bovis* genes previously linked by Sulyok et al. with AMR for various classes of antimicrobial, two sites linked with fluoroquinolone resistance (*gyrA* and *gyrB*) display multiple non-synonymous mutations (NSMs) for the high-MIC isolate 2019-043682 and no NSMs for the low-MIC isolate 1982-M6152. *ParC*, likewise associated with fluoroquinolone resistance, shows 18 unique NSMs in the isolate 2019-043682, and a single NSM in 1982-M6152, which is shared with the 2019-043682, therefore the shared single NSM is unlikely to be contributory to the elevated MICs. Although genes *rrs1-rrs2* and *rrl1-rrl2* were associated with AMR for tetracyclines, spectinomycin, macrolides, lincosamides and pleuromutilins, there are no NSMs for them in the isolate 2019-043682 despite the elevated MIC values, suggesting additional genetic events may be associated with AMR for these antimicrobials.

For antimicrobials where an observed increase in MIC was not matched with a previously identified *M. bovis* resistance-associated mutation, genes identified as AMR-associated in other species, as well as genes within the same functional groups are likely candidates for AMR association. Beyond the genes previously associated with AMR in *M. bovis*, an additional 510 features contain non-synonymous mutations. Assigning these genes to functional groups allowed us to exclude pseudogenes and genes coding for uncharacterized and hypothetical proteins. Also excluded were genes whose NSMs were identical between isolates 2019-043682 (high MIC) and 1982-M6152 (low MIC). Of the 149 genes remaining, we focused on a subset of 55 genes with nonsynonymous mutations within functional roles known to be involved in antimicrobial resistance [13]: protein synthesis and topoisomerases. Additionally, 22 genes with NSMs were identified as ATP binding cassette (ABC) transporter system genes. These genes, although lacking full characterization, are nonetheless included in the discussion as targets for future analysis, due to the role of efflux pumps, particularly ABC transporters, in AMR.

3.1. Protein Synthesis

Interference with protein synthesis is a primary method of action for the antimicrobials, with different antimicrobials interfering at different stages of synthesis, and at different locations within the ribosome complex.

3.1.1. Methyltransferases

RNA methyltransferases methylate specific bases within ribosomal RNA, altering the physical structure of binding sites and other active sites within the ribosomal subunits [16,29,30]. Mutations within the 16S RNA methyltransferase family are known to confer aminoglycoside resistance within other bacterial species [16], and five genes (*rsmA, rsmD, rsmH, rsmI* and MBOVPG45_RS02280, a 16S uracil methyltransferase) within isolate 2019-043682 contain NSMs not found in isolate 1982-M6152. The 23S methyltransferase *rlmA* has been associated with AMR for tylosin [29], and while *rlmA* is wildtype in isolate 2019-043682, the related 23S methyltransferases *rlmB, rlmD* and *rlmH* contain 5, 11 and 1 unique NSMs respectively. *RlmB* has also been identified as a potential site for AMR mutations based on an analysis of its structure [15], although no mutational studies have been conducted. For tRNA methyltransferases, *trmD* is implicated in multi-drug resistance [31]: it is wildtype in isolate 2019-043682, but two related tRNA methyltransferases (*trmB* and MBOVPG45_RS00465, a cytidine methyltransferase) contain NSMs, with *trmB* containing a gene disruption.

3.1.2. Ribosomal Proteins

Mutations in *rpsC* and *rpsJ*, components of the 30S ribosomal subunit, are known to confer tetracycline resistance [18,20]. *RpsC* contains a single NSM in isolate 2019-043682 that is unique from the two NSMs observed in isolate 1982-M6152, but *rpsJ* is wildtype in isolate 2019-043682 and contains a single NSM in isolate 1982-M6152 that is therefore unlikely to influence MIC values. *RpsB* and *rpsE* contain 3 and 2 NSMs in the 2019 isolate, with a single, separate NSM present for *rpsE* in the 1982 isolate: mutations in these genes have been linked with aminoglycoside resistance [17,19], Additionally, five other 30S ribosomal proteins (*rpsD, rpsG, rpsP, rpsS*, and *rbfA*) contain NSMs in isolate 2019-043682.

Of the 50S ribosomal proteins with observed NSMs, *rplD* and *rplV* have been previously associated with macrolide resistance in *Clostridium perfringens* and two *Campylobacter* species [22,23] with *rplD* containing ten separate NSMs in the isolate 2019-043682. The 50S subunit gene *rplC*, where mutation has been previously associated with pleuromutilin resistance [32], contains a single NSM in the 2019 isolate, unique from the two NSMs found in the 1982 isolate. 50S ribosomal proteins mutations have also been linked with resistance to lincosamides, macrolides and phenicols [32]: an additional five genes (*rplB, rpmE*, MBOVPG45_RS00445, MBOVPG45_RS03525 and MBOVPG45_RS01360) coding for 50S ribosomal proteins contain NSMs in isolate 2019-043682 while remaining wildtype in isolate 1982-M6152. Among these, *rpmE* has been linked with multi-drug resistance [24].

3.1.3. Aminoacyl-tRNA Synthetases

While none of the antimicrobials used in MIC testing in this study target them, aminoacyl-tRNA synthetases, also known as tRNA-ligases, are enzymes which attach individual amino acids to their corresponding tRNAs and are a target of interest for antimicrobial development [33]. Isolate 2019-043682 contains 22 tRNA-ligase genes with NSMs, of which ileS (a known target for pseudomonic acid) [27] is disrupted, as is alaS (a novobiocin target) [25], in addition to a glutamate-tRNA ligase (MBOVPG45_RSO1150) and a methionine-tRNA ligase (MBOVPG45_RS03150). *AsnS* and *pheS* have been linked with multi-drug resistance [26] and contain one and two unique NSMs in isolate 2019-043682, respectively. Three of these genes (alaS, ileS and MBOVPG45_RS02170, a threonine-tRNA ligase) contain different NSMs in isolate 1982-M6152, illustrating that the presence of an NSM on its own is not sufficient for AMR, and deeper investigation into changes in protein structure and function are required. LysS, containing 3 NSMs in isolate 2019-043682, has been identified as a gene contributing to methicillin resistance in MRSA [31]: as a β-lactam, methicillin is not used in the treatment of mycoplasma infections, but co-infection with *M. bovis* containing a potential AMR-associated mutation raises the possibility of horizontal gene transfer to a normally susceptible species.

3.2. Topoisomerases

In addition to *gyrA*, *gyrB* and *parC* discussed by Sulyok et al. (2017), *parE* mutations are also involved in fluoroquinolone resistance [14] and the isolate 2019-043682 contains four NSMs within the *parE* gene. While *topA*, a type I DNA topoisomerase, has not been linked with AMR previously, the gene, which is wildtype in isolate 1982-M6152, contains a single nucleotide "A" insertion at nt 1762 of the *topA* gene in isolate 2019-043682, which results in a *topA* (612–614 VK *) to *topA* (612–613 S *) mutation, likely a gene disrupting mutation. As bacterial topoisomerase I is a target of interest for antimicrobial development [34–36], screening for mutations affecting *topA* may be of future value to researchers and clinicians.

3.3. Bacterial Efflux Pumps: ABC Transporters

Bacterial efflux pumps are a class of membrane transport proteins whose role is the removal of toxic substances or metabolites from within the bacterial cell: It is estimated that 5–10% of all bacterial genes are involved in transport, with efflux pumps specifically comprising a large proportion of these transporters [37]. Of the two classes of efflux pump, primary and secondary, the primary transporters use ATP hydrolysis as an energy source, and are also known as ATP binding cassette transporters, or ABC transporters [38]. They are more commonly implicated in resistance to a single drug or category of drugs, although instances of multi-drug resistant ABC transporters have been described 200 [16,38].

As summarized in Table 4, 22 ABC transporter genes contain NSMs in isolate 2019-043682, one of which (MBOVPG45_RS03705) contains a gene-disrupting mutation. Three (MBOVPG45_RS01775, MBOVPG45_RS02905 and MBOVPG45_RS04315) also contain NSMs in isolate 1982-M6152. Although none are previously identified as SDR- or MDR- involved in *M. bovis*, the wide range of antimicrobials affected by efflux pumps suggests that this may be an area of interest for future research. While 8 non-ABC membrane transport proteins with NSMs were identified in isolate 2019-043682 (Supplementary Table S2), none has been characterized sufficiently to determine their potential as secondary efflux pumps and have thus been excluded from discussion.

3.4. Future Directions

Within the 55 genes selected for additional study based on functional role and the 22 ABC transporter genes, the 40 genes identified by their organism (eg., MBOVPG45_RS00380) rather than a common name limit the utility of a literature review or database search for assessing AMR potential. Although beyond the scope of the current study, a BLAST search for each gene to identify homology with other organisms could permit more detailed characterization of these genes and thus allow for a more thorough search of existing research into AMR. This would be of particular value for the ABC transporters, as all 22 identified as potential AMR associations due to their mutations are given *M. bovis*-specific identifiers. MBOVPG45_RS04315, with 89 separate NSMs in the high-MIC isolate, is a particularly strong candidate for a homology search.

As an initial foray by the research group into whole genome sequencing, the sequencing of a pair of high and low MIC isolates and the use of a fully-characterized reference strain (PG45) as a scaffold for assembly and annotation allowed us to determine which genes and which NSMs were non-contributory to the high MIC observed in the 2019 isolate, and allowed us to determine that no additional genes were present relative to the reference strain. Sequencing additional high-MIC strains of *M. bovis* as they arise in the future will allow us to develop further evidence in support of AMR association for the subset of genes identified and may uncover additional candidate genes for AMR association. Likewise, selecting historical strains for WGS that are high or low MIC for specific antimicrobials may allow for further refinement or expansion of the list of AMR-association candidates.

4. Materials and Methods

As a non-interventionary study, prior approval from the University of Guelph Research Ethics Board was not required for this research.

4.1. Culture & Isolation of Mycoplasmas

The body of a two-week old male Holstein calf was submitted to the Animal Health Lab in July of 2019 for post-mortem examination. Histologically, no lesions indicative of mycoplasma pneumonia were observed within the lungs. Culture and isolation of *M. bovis* AHL# 2019-043682 from the calf lung tissue was conducted as follows: The lung tissue submitted was perforated repeatedly using a sterile dry swab to collect sample material for broth (pig serum, horse serum and ureaplasma broths) and agar plate (pig serum agar, yeastolate agar, ureaplasma agar) culture [39]. Mycoplasma agar plates were incubated at 37 °C with 5–7% CO2 and 80–100% relative humidity. Ureaplasma agar plates ware incubated at 37 °C anaerobically. All broth cultures were incubated aerobically at 37 °C. Plates were read at 48–72 h intervals using a transilluminated stereomicroscope. Broth tubes were visually inspected for growth and pH change at 18–24 h intervals, and were subcultured twice, at 48–72 h growth and at 48–72 h following the first subculture. Agar plates were subcultured if suspicious growth was observed during reading. Following isolation, species identity as *M bovis* was confirmed using goat anti-rabbit/fluorescein isothiocyanate (GAR/FITC)-labelled antiserum fluorescent antibody staining [39]. Blocks of agar containing pure isolate were cut and stored at −80 °C for long term storage. Isolated 1982-M6152, an isolate of *M. bovis* from 1982 stored at −80 °C and identified in a previous study [3] as low MIC for most antimicrobials, was propagated and tested by WGS and MIC retesting.

4.2. MIC Testing

Minimum inhibitory concentration (MIC) testing was conducted on *M. bovis* isolates 2019-043682, 1982-M6152 and strain PG45 in triplicates for each isolate using previously described procedures [3], and using *M. bovis* isolate 227, an internal laboratory reference strain, as a control. Briefly: each isolate was first inoculated into 4 mL Mycoplasma MIC broth and incubated 48–72 h at 37 °C aerobically, before being frozen at −80 °C.

Following this incubation period, a colour-changing unit (CCU) and colony forming unit (CFU) count were setup to determine the number of CCU's in the frozen aliquots. A 10-fold serial dilution was prepared for each isolate using Mycoplasma MIC broth, with 200 µL total volume in each of 12 wells. 10µL of the first 6 dilutions were plated onto Hayflick's agar, and both the serial dilutions and agar plates were incubated for 48–72 h at 37 °C with 5–7% CO_2 and 80–100% relative humidity. Both serial dilutions (lowest serial dilution showing a blue-red colour change) and agar plates (colonies counted using a stereomicroscope) were read after 48–72 h, and the CCU and CFU counts of the isolates were calculated accordingly.

A frozen aliquot was thawed and diluted in tubes of Mycoplasma MIC broth in successively larger volumes so that at least 25 mL of a 103–105 CCU/mL dilution was achieved. MIC testing was setup by inoculating 200 μL of this dilution into every well of a Sensititre BOPO6F microtitre plate. The Sensititre plate was incubated at 37 °C with 5–7% CO_2 and 80–100% relative humidity for 24–72 h, until the positive control wells showed a blue-red colour change. At this point the Sensititre plate was read, and any wells showing a blue-red colour change were noted. The MIC for each antibiotic was calculated as the lowest concentration of drug that suppressed growth. After the Sensititre plate had been inoculated, the CCU and CFU counts of the inoculum were determined as previously described.

4.3. Nucleic Acid Extraction

For the isolates 1982-M6152, 2019-043682 and *M. bovis* PG45, 100 μL of a broth culture was extracted on the Applied Biosystems MagMAX 96 automated nucleic acid extraction platform (Applied Biosystems, Foster City, CA, USA) using the Low Cell Content protocol for the MagMAX Pathogen DNA/RNA kit (Applied Biosystems). Samples were eluted in a final volume of 90 μL, using the elution buffer provided with the kit, then held at −20 °C until prepared for WGS.

4.4. Whole Genome Sequencing & Bioinformatics

A 2 × 251 paired end sequencing reaction was conducted on the Illumina MiSeq platform (Illumina, San Diego, CA, USA) using a Nextera XT kit (Illumina) and associated protocols for whole genome sequencing (Illumina Custom Protocol Selector, Illumina Inc.) Quality filtering and assembly of FASTQ files was done on instrument and then uploaded to Illumina's BaseSpace storage and computing cloud. On BaseSpace, genome assembly was conducted using SPAdes Genome Assembler v3.9.0 [11], and MLST assignment of two isolates using the Bacterial Analysis Pipeline v1.0.4 [12].

The assembled FASTQ files were then downloaded from BaseSpace, the adapter for the Nextera XT Kit (CTGTCTCTTATACACATCT) trimmed, then the genomes were assembled using bioinformatics software DNAstar (V17) (DNASTAR, Madison, WI, USA) using NGS-Based Reference-guide (small genomes, contigs) of Hybrid reference-guide/de novo genome assembly function against and annotated with features from reference genome *M. bovis* PG45 (GenBank Accession: NC_014760.1). Multiple genome alignment was performed using Mauve Genome of Geneious v11 (Auckland, New Zealand) with automatically calculated seed weight and automatically calculated minimum LCB score. SNPs were analyzed with MegAlign, DNASTAR's ArrayStar v14 (DNASTAR, Madison, WI, USA), and Geneious v11 to identify deleted and truncated genes, SNPs and non-synonymous mutations relative to *M. bovis* PG45. Gene features were then tabulated in a spreadsheet (Supplementary Table S2) and further annotated by searching NCBI's Gene database to identify their functional roles where possible. Named genes with functional roles in protein synthesis and topoisomerase structure that contained NSMs or disruptions in the 2019 isolate were selected for additional study, using the CARD database [13] and literature review (Google Scholar, keywords used: "antimicrobial resistance", "antibiotic resistance", AMR, and the gene name or functional group, I.e. "rplD" "antimicrobial resistance") to identify mechanisms of antimicrobial resistance, and *M. bovis* gene homologues with AMR association in other organisms.

5. Conclusions

This study identified 55 genetic events of nonsynonymous mutations and gene disruptions linked to *M. bovis* AMR. Future studies are warranted to further analyze these candidate genes, identifying the effects of the altered amino acids on protein structure and their link to AMR. Additionally, mutated genes identified in this study but currently uncharacterized may be assigned to functional groups in future.

Supplementary Materials: The following are available online at http://www.mdpi.com/2076-0817/9/7/588/s1, Table S1: ArrayStar Output of Nonsynonymous Mutations, Table S2: Summary of NSMs, Table S3: AMR-Associated Gene Candidates. WGS sequence data for 1982-M6152 (Accession: CP058969) and 2019-043682 (Accession: CP058968) are available through GenBank.

Author Contributions: Contributor roles for this publication are defined as follows: Conceptualization, H.Y.C; methodology, H.Y.C., J.E. and L.L.; software, H.Y.C.; validation, H.Y.C., L.L., J.E.; formal analysis, H.Y.C. and L.L.; investigation, J.E. and L.L.; resources, H.Y.C.; data curation, H.Y.C. and L.L.; writing—original draft preparation, L.L.; writing—review and editing, H.Y.C. and J.E.; visualization, L.L., H.Y.C.; supervision, H.Y.C.; project administration, H.Y.C.; funding acquisition, H.Y.C. All authors have read and agreed to the published version of the manuscript.

Funding: This study was supported in part by the Ontario Animal Health Network, funded by the University of Guelph-OMAFRA Partnership Agreement and the Animal Health Laboratory (AHL), University of Guelph, Canada.

Acknowledgments: We greatly appreciate the technical support and advice on Illumina BaseSpace software provided by Aparna Krishnamurthy and Durda Slavic, Animal Health Laboratory, University of Guelph, Canada.

Conflicts of Interest: The authors declare no conflict of interest. The funders had no role in the design of the study; in the collection, analyses, or interpretation of data; in the writing of the manuscript, or in the decision to publish the results.

References

1. Caswell, J.L.; Bateman, K.G.; Cai, H.Y.; Castillo-Alcala, F. Mycoplasma bovis in Respiratory Disease of Feedlot Cattle. *Vet. Clin. N. Am. Food Anim. Pract.* **2010**, *26*, 365–379. [CrossRef]
2. Griffin, D.; Chengappa, M.M.; Kuszak, J.; McVey, D.S. Bacterial Pathogens of the Bovine Respiratory Disease Complex. *Vet. Clin. N. Am. Food Anim. Pract.* **2010**, *26*, 381–394. [CrossRef]
3. Cai, H.Y.; McDowall, R.; Parker, L.; Kaufman, E.I.; Caswell, J.L. Changes in antimicrobial susceptibility profiles of Mycoplasma bovis over time. *Can. J. Vet. Res.* **2019**, *83*, 34–41.
4. Byrne, W.J.; McCormack, R.; Egan, J.; Brice, N.; Ball, H.J.; Markey, B. Isolation of Mycoplasma bovis from bovine clinical samples in the Republic of Ireland. *Vet. Rec.* **2001**, *148*, 331–333. [CrossRef]
5. Rosenbusch, R.F.; Kinyon, J.M.; Apley, M.; Funk, N.D.; Smith, S.; Hoffman, L.J. In Vitro Antimicrobial Inhibition Profiles of Mycoplasma Bovis Isolates Recovered from Various Regions of the United States from 2002 to 2003. *J. Vet. Diagn. Investig.* **2005**, *17*, 436–441. [CrossRef]
6. Lysnyansky, I.; Ayling, R.D. Mycoplasma bovis: Mechanisms of Resistance and Trends in Antimicrobial Susceptibility. *Front. Microbiol.* **2016**, *7*, 595. [CrossRef]
7. Baym, M.; Stone, L.K.; Kishony, R. Multidrug evolutionary strategies to reverse antibiotic resistance. *Science* **2016**, *351*, aad3292. [CrossRef] [PubMed]
8. Owen, J.R.; Noyes, N.; Young, A.E.; Prince, D.J.; Blanchard, P.C.; Lehenbauer, T.W.; Aly, S.S.; Davis, J.H.; O'Rourke, S.M.; Abdo, Z.; et al. Whole-Genome Sequencing and Concordance Between Antimicrobial Susceptibility Genotypes and Phenotypes of Bacterial Isolates Associated with Bovine Respiratory Disease. *G3 Genes Genomes Genet.* **2017**, *7*, 3059–3071. [CrossRef] [PubMed]
9. Sulyok, K.M.; Kreizinger, Z.; Wehmann, E.; Lysnyansky, I.; Bányai, K.; Marton, S.; Jerzsele, Á.; Rónai, Z.; Turcsányi, I.; Makrai, L.; et al. Mutations Associated with Decreased Susceptibility to Seven Antimicrobial Families in Field and Laboratory-Derived Mycoplasma bovis Strains. *Antimicrob. Agents Chemother.* **2017**, *61*. [CrossRef] [PubMed]
10. Sato, T.; Higuchi, H.; Yokota, S.; Tamura, Y. Mycoplasma bovis isolates from dairy calves in Japan have less susceptibility than a reference strain to all approved macrolides associated with a point mutation (G748A) combined with multiple species-specific nucleotide alterations in 23S rRNA. *Microbiol. Immunol.* **2017**, *61*, 215–224. [CrossRef] [PubMed]
11. Nurk, S.; Bankevich, A.; Antipov, D.; Gurevich, A.; Korobeynikov, A.; Lapidus, A.; Prjibelsky, A.; Pyshkin, A.; Sirotkin, A.; Sirotkin, Y.; et al. Assembling Genomes and Mini-metagenomes from Highly Chimeric Reads. In *Proc Research Comp Molecular Bio*; Deng, M., Jiang, R., Sun, F., Zhang, X., Eds.; Springer: Berlin/ Heidelberg, Germany, 2013; pp. 158–170.
12. Thomsen, M.C.F.; Ahrenfeldt, J.; Cisneros, J.L.B.; Jurtz, V.; Larsen, M.V.; Hasman, H.; Aarestrup, F.M.; Lund, O. A Bacterial Analysis Platform: An Integrated System for Analysing Bacterial Whole Genome Sequencing Data for Clinical Diagnostics and Surveillance. *PLoS ONE* **2016**, *11*, e0157718. [CrossRef] [PubMed]

13. Alcock, B.P.; Raphenya, A.R.; Lau, T.T.Y.; Tsang, K.K.; Bouchard, M.; Edalatmand, A.; Huynh, W.; Nguyen, A.-L.V.; Cheng, A.A.; Liu, S.; et al. CARD 2020: antibiotic resistome surveillance with the comprehensive antibiotic resistance database. *Nucleic Acids Res.* **2020**, *48*, D517–D525. [CrossRef] [PubMed]
14. Perichon, B.; Tankovic, J.; Courvalin, P. Characterization of a mutation in the parE gene that confers fluoroquinolone resistance in Streptococcus pneumoniae. *Antimicrob. Agents Chemother.* **1997**, *41*, 1166–1167. [CrossRef]
15. Michel, G.; Sauvé, V.; Larocque, R.; Li, Y.; Matte, A.; Cygler, M. The Structure of the RlmB 23S rRNA Methyltransferase Reveals a New Methyltransferase Fold with a Unique Knot. *Structure* **2002**, *10*, 1303–1315. [CrossRef]
16. Fyfe, C.; Grossman, T.H.; Kerstein, K.; Sutcliffe, J. Resistance to Macrolide Antibiotics in Public Health Pathogens. *Cold Spring Harb. Perspect. Med.* **2016**, *6*, a025395. [CrossRef] [PubMed]
17. Feng, Y.; Jonker, M.J.; Moustakas, I.; Brul, S.; Ter Kuile, B.H. Dynamics of Mutations during Development of Resistance by Pseudomonas aeruginosa against Five Antibiotics. *Antimicrob. Agents Chemother.* **2016**, *60*, 4229–4236. [CrossRef]
18. Grossman, T.H. Tetracycline Antibiotics and Resistance. *Cold Spring Harb. Perspect. Med.* **2016**, *6*, a025387. [CrossRef]
19. Wang, Z.; Kong, L.C.; Jia, B.Y.; Liu, S.M.; Jiang, X.Y.; Ma, H.X. Aminoglycoside susceptibility of Pasteurella multocida isolates from bovine respiratory infections in China and mutations in ribosomal protein S5 associated with high-level induced spectinomycin resistance. *J. Vet. Med. Sci.* **2017**, *79*, 1678–1681. [CrossRef]
20. Hu, M.; Nandi, S.; Davies, C.; Nicholas, R.A. High-Level Chromosomally Mediated Tetracycline Resistance in Neisseria gonorrhoeae Results from a Point Mutation in the rpsJ Gene Encoding Ribosomal Protein S10 in Combination with the mtrR and penB Resistance Determinants. *Antimicrob. Agents Chemother.* **2005**, *49*, 4327–4334. [CrossRef]
21. Long, K.S.; Hansen, L.H.; Jakobsen, L.; Vester, B. Interaction of Pleuromutilin Derivatives with the Ribosomal Peptidyl Transferase Center. *Antimicrob. Agents Chemother.* **2006**, *50*, 1458–1462. [CrossRef]
22. Hölzel, C.S.; Harms, K.S.; Schwaiger, K.; Bauer, J. Resistance to Linezolid in a Porcine Clostridium perfringens Strain Carrying a Mutation in the rplD Gene Encoding the Ribosomal Protein L4. *Antimicrob. Agents Chemother.* **2010**, *54*, 1351–1353. [CrossRef] [PubMed]
23. Cagliero, C.; Mouline, C.; Cloeckaert, A.; Payot, S. Synergy between Efflux Pump CmeABC and Modifications in Ribosomal Proteins L4 and L22 in Conferring Macrolide Resistance in Campylobacter jejuni and Campylobacter coli. *Antimicrob. Agents Chemother.* **2006**, *50*, 3893–3896. [CrossRef] [PubMed]
24. Liu, A.; Tran, L.; Becket, E.; Lee, K.; Chinn, L.; Park, E.; Tran, K.; Miller, J.H. Antibiotic Sensitivity Profiles Determined with an Escherichia coli Gene Knockout Collection: Generating an Antibiotic Bar Code. *Antimicrob. Agents Chemother.* **2010**, *54*, 1393–1403. [CrossRef] [PubMed]
25. Milija, J.; Lilic, M.; Janjusevic, R.; Jovanovic, G.; Savic, D.J. tRNA Synthetase Mutants of Escherichia coli K-12 Are Resistant to the Gyrase Inhibitor Novobiocin. *J. Bacteriol.* **1999**, *181*, 2979–2983. [CrossRef]
26. Magalhães, S.; Aroso, M.; Roxo, I.; Ferreira, S.; Cerveira, F.; Ramalheira, E.; Ferreira, R.; Vitorino, R. Proteomic profile of susceptible and multidrug-resistant clinical isolates of Escherichia coli and Klebsiella pneumoniae using label-free and immunoproteomic strategies. *Res. Microbiol.* **2017**, *168*, 222–233. [CrossRef] [PubMed]
27. Yanagisawa, T.; Lee, J.T.; Wu, H.C.; Kawakami, M. Relationship of protein structure of isoleucyl-tRNA synthetase with pseudomonic acid resistance of Escherichia coli. A proposed mod of action of pseudomonic acid as an inhibitor of isoleucyl-tRNA synthetase. *J. Biol. Chem.* **1994**, *269*, 24304–24309.
28. Dordel, J.; Kim, C.; Chung, M.; Pardos de la Gándara, M.; Holden, M.T.J.; Parkhill, J.; de Lencastre, H.; Bentley, S.D.; Tomasz, A. Novel Determinants of Antibiotic Resistance: Identification of Mutated Loci in Highly Methicillin-Resistant Subpopulations of Methicillin-Resistant Staphylococcus aureus. *MBio* **2014**, *5*. [CrossRef]
29. Liu, M.; Douthwaite, S. Resistance to the macrolide antibiotic tylosin is conferred by single methylations at 23S rRNA nucleotides G748 and A2058 acting in synergy. *Proc. Natl. Acad. Sci. USA* **2002**, *99*, 14658–14663. [CrossRef]
30. Doi, Y.; Arakawa, Y. 16S Ribosomal RNA Methylation: Emerging Resistance Mechanism against Aminoglycosides. *Clin. Infect. Dis.* **2007**, *45*, 88–94. [CrossRef]

31. Masuda, I.; Matsubara, R.; Christian, T.; Rojas, E.R.; Yadavalli, S.S.; Zhang, L.; Goulian, M.; Foster, L.J.; Huang, K.C.; Hou, Y.-M. tRNA Methylation Is a Global Determinant of Bacterial Multi-drug Resistance. *Cell Syst.* **2019**, *8*, 302–314. [CrossRef]
32. Giguère, S. Lincosamides, Pleuromutilins, and Streptogramins. In *Antimicrobial Therapy in Veterinary Medicine*; John Wiley & Sons Ltd: Hoboken, NJ, USA, 2013; pp. 199–210. ISBN 978-1-118-67501-4.
33. Hurdle, J.G.; O'Neill, A.J.; Chopra, I. Prospects for Aminoacyl-tRNA Synthetase Inhibitors as New Antimicrobial Agents. *Antimicrob. Agents Chemother.* **2005**, *49*, 4821–4833. [CrossRef] [PubMed]
34. Tse-Dinh, Y.-C. Bacterial topoisomerase I as a target for discovery of antibacterial compounds. *Nucleic Acids Res.* **2009**, *37*, 731–737. [CrossRef] [PubMed]
35. Bansal, S.; Tawar, U.; Singh, M.; Nikravesh, A.; Good, L.; Tandon, V. Old class but new dimethoxy analogue of benzimidazole: A bacterial topoisomerase I inhibitor. *Int. J. Antimicrob. Agents* **2010**, *35*, 186–190. [CrossRef] [PubMed]
36. Nagaraja, V.; Godbole, A.A.; Henderson, S.R.; Maxwell, A. DNA topoisomerase I and DNA gyrase as targets for TB therapy. *Drug Discov. Today* **2017**, *22*, 510–518. [CrossRef]
37. Webber, M.A.; Piddock, L.J.V. The importance of efflux pumps in bacterial antibiotic resistance. *J Antimicrob. Chemother.* **2003**, *51*, 9–11. [CrossRef]
38. Marquez, B. Bacterial efflux systems and efflux pumps inhibitors. *Biochimie* **2005**, *87*, 1137–1147. [CrossRef]
39. Ruhnke, H.L.; Rosendal, S. Useful Protocols for Diagnosis of Animal Mycoplasmas. In *Mycoplasmosis in Animals: Laboratory Diagnosis*; Whitford, H.W., Rosenbusch, R.F., Lauerman, L.H., Eds.; Iowa State University Press: Ames, IA, USA, 1994; pp. 141–166.

pathogens

MDPI

Article

Investigation of Macrolide Resistance Genotypes in *Mycoplasma bovis* Isolates from Canadian Feedlot Cattle

Andrea Kinnear [1], Tim A. McAllister [2], Rahat Zaheer [2], Matthew Waldner [1], Antonio C. Ruzzini [1,3], Sara Andrés-Lasheras [2], Sarah Parker [1], Janet E. Hill [1] and Murray D. Jelinski [1,*]

1 Western College of Veterinary Medicine, University of Saskatchewan, Saskatoon, SK S7N 5B4, Canada; andrea.kinnear@usask.ca (A.K.); matthew.waldner@usask.ca (M.W.); antonio.ruzzini@usask.ca (A.C.R.); sarah.parker@usask.ca (S.P.); janet.hill@usask.ca (J.E.H.)

2 Lethbridge Research and Development Centre, Agriculture and Agri-Food Canada, Lethbridge, AB T1J 4B1, Canada; tim.mcallister@canada.ca (T.A.M.); rahat.zaheer@canada.ca (R.Z.); sara.andreslasheras@canada.ca (S.A.-L.)

3 College of Medicine, Department of Biochemistry, Microbiology and Immunology, University of Saskatchewan, Saskatoon, SK S7N 5E5, Canada

* Correspondence: murray.jelinski@usask.ca; Tel.: +1-306-966-7166

Received: 30 June 2020; Accepted: 28 July 2020; Published: 30 July 2020

Abstract: *Mycoplasma bovis* is associated with bovine respiratory disease (BRD) and chronic pneumonia and polyarthritis syndrome (CPPS) in feedlot cattle. No efficacious vaccines for *M. bovis* exist; hence, macrolides are commonly used to control mycoplasmosis. Whole genome sequences of 126 *M. bovis* isolates, derived from 96 feedlot cattle over 12 production years, were determined. Antimicrobial susceptibility testing (AST) of five macrolides (gamithromycin, tildipirosin, tilmicosin, tulathromycin, tylosin) was conducted using a microbroth dilution method. The AST phenotypes were compared to the genotypes generated for 23S rRNA and the L4 and L22 ribosomal proteins. Mutations in domains II (nucleotide 748; *E. coli* numbering) and V (nucleotide 2059 and 2060) of the 23S rRNA (*rrl*) gene alleles were associated with resistance. All isolates with a single mutation at Δ748 were susceptible to tulathromycin, but resistant to tilmicosin and tildipirosin. Isolates with mutations in both domain II and V (Δ748Δ2059 or Δ748Δ2060) were resistant to all five macrolides. However, >99% of isolates were resistant to tildipirosin and tilmicosin, regardless of the number and positions of the mutations. Isolates with a Δ748 mutation in the 23S rRNA gene and mutations in L4 and L22 were resistant to all macrolides except for tulathromycin.

Keywords: antimicrobial; susceptibility; resistance; genotype; rRNA; macrolides; feedlot; beef; cattle

1. Introduction

Mycoplasma bovis is associated with various diseases of cattle such as pneumonia, mastitis, arthritis, otitis media, conjunctivitis, and reproductive disorders [1,2]. In feedlot cattle, *M. bovis* infections commonly manifest as bovine respiratory disease (BRD) and chronic pneumonia and polyarthritis syndrome (CPPS) [3,4]. Furthermore, *M. bovis* infections often respond poorly to antimicrobial therapy, resulting in a chronic infection [5]. This lack of a response frequently results in prolonged antimicrobial therapy, which indiscriminately selects for antimicrobial resistance in the pathogens that comprise the BRD complex [6]. Mycoplasmosis in the feedlot results in economic losses due to reduced production performance, increased treatment costs, and death loss [2,6]. In addition, feedlot cattle with polyarthritis may become severely lame, which is a significant animal welfare issue.

As there are currently no effective vaccines for *M. bovis*, antimicrobials remain the primary means for the prevention and control of mycoplasmosis [2,7]. This has led to a number of *M. bovis* antimicrobial susceptibility studies in Canada [8–11], United States [12], Japan [13] and Europe [7,14–19]. These studies suggest that *M. bovis* will continue to become increasingly resistant to antimicrobials. This situation is exacerbated by the limited number of antimicrobials available for treating mycoplasma infections. *Mycoplasma* spp. lack a cell wall and the ability to synthesize folate, rendering them intrinsically resistant to all β-lactams and sulfonamides [2]. In addition, most aminoglycosides either lack label claims for BRD, or the formulations are not amenable for use in feedlot cattle. This narrows the selection of antimicrobials to those that target protein synthesis or DNA replication, and that have been formulated to maintain therapeutic blood levels for several days. The main class of antimicrobials that meet these criteria is the macrolides.

Macrolides have been formulated to be administered parenterally or in-feed; however, only one macrolide, tylosin tartrate (TYLT), is registered in Canada for in-feed use. Tylosin is typically administered throughout the feeding period, and is used to control liver abscesses [9]. The other four main macrolides used in the feedlot are: tilmicosin (TIL), tildipirosin (TIP), tulathromycin (TUL), and gamithromycin (GAM). All of which are formulated as long-acting injectable antimicrobials, and depending on the drug, may have label claims for the control (metaphylaxis) and treatment of BRD. A distinctive pharmacological characteristic of macrolides that makes them ideally suited for use in feedlot cattle is their predilection to concentrate in the pulmonary epithelial fluid [20]. This is notable because BRD is the most prevalent and costly disease of feedlot cattle [21]. Thus, the macrolides' pharmacokinetic and pharmacodynamic profiles are particularly well suited for metaphylaxis therapy for BRD in feedlots [22]. In western Canada, cattle deemed to be a high risk for developing BRD often receive TUL at the time of arrival to the feedlot; whereas, low risk cattle may receive either no antimicrobials or a long-acting oxytetracycline [23]. Lastly, unlike other BRD pathogens, antimicrobial resistance in *M. bovis* is not associated with antimicrobial resistance genes [24], but rather resistance arises from mutations in ribosomal RNAs [25].

Macrolides are a member of the macrolide–lincosamide–streptogramin B (MLS_B) superfamily, all of which exert a bacteriostatic effect by disrupting protein synthesis [26]. Specifically, they bind with domains II and V of 23S rRNA, which is a component of 50S ribosomal subunit [27,28]. Ribosomal proteins L4 and L22 are positioned in close proximity to these macrolide binding sites [28,29]. Mutations within 23S rRNA and the L4 and L22 ribosomal proteins are associated with macrolide resistance [25,30]. This mechanism of resistance is not unique to *M. bovis* [13,31,32], having been reported in a variety of bacterial species, including other *Mycoplasma* spp. [33,34], *Neisseria gonorrhoeae* [30], *Streptococcus* spp. [35,36], *Francisella tularensis* [37], *Escherichia coli* [38], *Chlamydia trachomatis* [39], and *Haemophilus influenzae* [40].

A limitation of antimicrobial susceptibility testing (AST) for *M. bovis* is the lack of established clinical breakpoints from the Clinical and Laboratory Standards Institute (CLSI) and the European Committee on Antimicrobial Susceptibility Testing (EUCAST). As a result, researchers have extrapolated *M. bovis* clinical breakpoints from human *Mycoplasma* spp. and other bovine respiratory pathogens for which clinical breakpoints have been established [9,11,12,15,41–43]. Another challenge with performing AST on *M. bovis* is its very fastidious culture requirements, which is related to its reduced genome and limited biosynthetic capacity [44]. These requirements, coupled with relatively slow nonprolific growth, have encouraged the development of rapid molecular testing techniques for predicting antimicrobial susceptibility for *M. bovis* [13,45]. Utilization of a genotypic approach to assess antimicrobial susceptibility of *M. bovis* could allow for more expeditious evaluation of antimicrobial efficacy and evidence-based selection of antimicrobials to enable judicious use of antimicrobials, which are all principles of antimicrobial stewardship. Additionally, a genotypic approach could be more amenable as a standardized approach to assess antimicrobial susceptibility in *M. bovis* than culture-based techniques, as it would not be susceptible to variable results due to growth conditions. To support these efforts, this study assessed the concordance between genotypes known to confer macrolide resistance to AST phenotypes. Specifically, the study compared the 23S rRNA, L4, and L22 genotypes of *M. bovis* isolates to the AST results of five macrolides commonly used in western Canadian feedlot cattle to control and treat BRD.

2. Results

2.1. Culture and Reference Antimicrobial Susceptibilities

A total of 126 *Mycoplasma bovis* isolates were derived from 96 head of feedlot cattle from 21 feedlots over 12 production years, 2006 to 2018 (Table 1). Thirty head of cattle provided paired lung/joint isolates (n = 60), 14 provided a lung sample, 5 provided a joint isolate, and 47 isolates came from the nasopharynx. Nasopharyngeal isolates were derived from healthy (n = 30), diseased (n = 15), and dead (n = 2) cattle. Phenotypically resistant isolates to the macrolides tested were derived from samples taken from healthy, diseased, and dead cattle (Table 2). Production years were used to define the sampling cohort, as animals often enter the feedlot in the fall and remain until the following calendar year. Thus, the 2018 production year included samples obtained between 1 November 2018 and 30 June 2019.

Table 1. *Mycoplasma bovis* isolates (n = 126) by anatomical location, health status, and production year.

	Production Year								
	2006	2007	2008	2014	2015	2016	2017	2018	Total
Anatomical Location									
Joint		1	1	1	1	14	11	6	35
Lung				3	3	17	15	6	44
Nasopharynx	5	28					9	5	47
Total	5	29	1	4	4	31	35	17	126
Health Status									
Healthy	2	14					9	5	30
Diseased	3	12							15
Dead		3	1	4	4	31	26	12	81
Total	5	29	1	4	4	31	35	17	126

Table 2. Number of *Mycoplasma bovis* isolates (n = 126) with a resistant (R) or susceptible (S) phenotype by health status.

Health Status		Phenotype (% Resistant)					Total
		GAM	TIL	TIP	TUL	TYLT	
Healthy	R/S (%R)	19/11 (63.3)	30/0 (100)	30/0 (100)	11/19 (36.7)	22/8 (73.3)	30
Diseased	R/S (%R)	9/6 (60.0)	15/0 (100)	15/0 (100)	9/6 (60.0)	11/4 (73.3)	15
Dead	R/S (%R)	78/3 (96.3)	80/1 (98.8)	81/0 (100)	72/9 (88.9)	78/3 (96.3)	81
Total	R/S (%R)	106/20 (84.1)	125/1 (99.2)	126/0 (100)	92/34 (73.0)	111/15 (88.1)	126

GAM—gamithromycin, TIL—tilmicosin, TIP—tildipirosin, TUL—tulathromycin, and TYLT—tylosin.

Mycoplasma bovis PG45 (*Mycoplasma bovis* ATCC® 25523) was resequenced and possessed the equivalent 23S rRNA genotype at positions 748, 2059, and 2060, as reported in the published reference genome [46]. Compared to the published reference genome, no nonsynonymous mutations in L4 and L22 ribosomal proteins were observed in this resequenced isolate. The following minimum inhibitory concentration (MIC) values, defined as the lowest concentration of antimicrobial to visibly inhibit growth, were determined from AST of five PG45 replicates: GAM, 8–16; TIP, 4–8; TIL, 1; TUL,

0.25; and TYLT, 1–2 μg/mL. Due to these genotypic and phenotypic findings, *M. bovis* PG45 was considered to be a susceptible wildtype isolate.

2.2. Genome Sequencing and Assembly

Draft genomes of the 126 isolates were assembled from an average 210,113 paired reads (range: 55,951 to 414,042); average read length of 217 bp (range: 166 to 233 bp). This produced assemblies with an average N50 of 18,690 bp (range: 1780 to 34,113 bp), an average coverage depth of 45.3 (range 12.2 to 89.1), and an average of 579 contigs (range: 171 to 1639).

2.3. 23 S rRNA Gene

Among the 126 isolates analyzed, mutations (single nucleotide polymorphisms, SNPs) were located in hairpin 35 of domain II (nucleotide 748; *E. coli* numbering used throughout) and the peptidyl transferase loop of domain V (nucleotide 2059 and 2060) of the 23S rRNA (*rrl*) gene alleles. The 23S rRNA genotype was assigned based on alleles observed at position 748, 2059, and 2060 (Table 3). As there are up to two copies of the *rrl* gene reported for *M. bovis*, an isolate was categorized as having a change (Δ) if a mutation occurred in at least one copy of the gene. The *M. bovis* PG45 reference genome was considered as the reference (wildtype) and two isolates (1.6%) were identical to this 23S rRNA genotype. Most isolates (73.0%; 92/126) had mutations in domains II and V (Δ748Δ2059 or Δ748Δ2060); whereas, 25.4% (32/126) had a single mutation in domain II (Δ748). There were no isolates with lone mutations in domain V. All isolates with a single mutation at Δ748 were susceptible to TUL (MIC ≤ 16 μg/mL); resistant to TIP and TIL (MIC ≥ 8 μg/mL); and either susceptible (MIC ≤ 4 μg/mL) or resistant (MIC ≥ 8 μg/mL) to GAM and TYLT (Figure 1a). Isolates that had accumulated mutations in both domain II and V (Δ748Δ2059 or Δ748 Δ2060) were resistant to all five macrolides (Table 3 and Figure 1b).

No dose dependent effect was apparent within a given genotype (i.e., Δ748 only) for those with a single mutant allele (i.e., G748A) or a combined mutant/wildtype allele (i.e., G748, G748A). The MIC values for isolates with Δ748 only 23S rRNA genotype, with a single mutant allele, ranged from 1 to 128 μg/mL for GAM and TYLT, and 0.25 to 8 μg/mL for TUL. Isolates with combined alleles had consistently lower MIC values of 8, 8–16, and 0.25 μg/mL for GAM, TYLT, and TUL, respectively, which were within the MIC range for isolates with a single mutant allele. For isolates with the Δ748Δ2059 23S rRNA genotype, those with combined alleles had MIC values ranging from 8 to ≥128 μg/mL for TYLT compared to ≥128 μg/mL with a single mutant allele. Regardless of allelic composition, the MIC values for isolates with Δ748Δ2060 23S rRNA genotypes were ≥64 μg/mL.

The 23S rRNA genotypes were grouped based on the presence of mutations in domain II only versus domain II and V. The results were reported as % resistant with 95% confidence interval (95% CI) for a proportion (Table 4). The two isolates with wildtype 23S rRNA genotypes were susceptible to TUL and TYLT (0, 0–0.66), and 1 of 2 were resistant to GAM and TIL (0.5, 0.09–0.91). Isolates with mutations in domain II only (Δ748 only) had a similar proportion of isolates resistant to GAM (0.41, 0.26–0.58) and TYLT (0.59, 0.42–0.74) compared to TUL (0, 0–0.11). An additional mutation in domain V at positions 2059 (Δ748Δ2059) or 2060 (Δ748Δ2060) resulted in all isolates being resistant to all five macrolides. All isolates were resistant TIP, regardless of genotype.

Table 3. Comparison of 23S rRNA genotypes and the number (%) of *Mycoplasma bovis* isolates (n = 126) resistant to the five macrolides tested.

Genotype	23S rRNA Gene Alleles⁺ Domain II	Domain V		Percent (n) of Isolates	Phenotype# (% Resistant)				
	748	2059	2060		GAM	TIL	TIP	TUL	TYLT
Wildtype*	G748	A2059	A2060	1.6 (2)	1 (50)	1 (50)	2 (100)	0 (0)	0 (0)
	Total			1.6 (2)	1 (50)	1 (50)	2 (100)	0 (0)	0 (0)
Δ748 only	G748, G748A‡			4.0 (5)	5 (100)	5 (100)	5 (100)	0 (0)	5 (100)
	G748A			21.4 (27)	8 (29.6)	27 (100)	27 (100)	0 (0)	14 (51.9)
	Total			25.4 (32)	13 (40.6)	32 (100)	32 (100)	0 (0)	19 (59.4)
Δ748Δ2059	G748, G748A‡	A2059, A2059G‡		0.8 (1)	1 (100)	1 (100)	1 (100)	1 (100)	1 (100)
	G748A	A2059, A2059G‡		2.4 (3)	3 (100)	3 (100)	3 (100)	3 (100)	3 (100)
	G748A	A2059, A2059C‡		2.4 (3)	3 (100)	3 (100)	3 (100)	3 (100)	3 (100)
	G748A	A2059, A2059T‡		7.1 (9)	9 (100)	9 (100)	9 (100)	9 (100)	9 (100)
	G748A	A2059G		49.2 (62)	62 (100)	62 (100)	62 (100)	62 (100)	62 (100)
	Total			61.9 (78)	78 (100)	78 (100)	78 (100)	78 (100)	78 (100)
Δ748Δ2060	G748A		A2060, A2060C‡	0.8 (1)	1 (100)	1 (100)	1 (100)	1 (100)	1 (100)
	G748A		A2060C	7.9 (10)	10 (100)	10 (100)	10 (100)	10 (100)	10 (100)
	G748A		A2060G	2.4 (3)	3 (100)	3 (100)	3 (100)	3 (100)	3 (100)
	Total			11.1 (14)	14 (100)	14 (100)	14 (100)	14 (100)	14 (100)

* *Mycoplasma bovis* PG45 is designated as wildtype genotype. # GAM—gamithromycin, TIL—tilmicosin, TIP—tildipirosin, TUL—tulathromycin, and TYLT—tylosin. ‡ Representative of a combined wildtype and mutant allele. ⁺ Positioning of the alleles is based on *Escherichia coli* numbering.

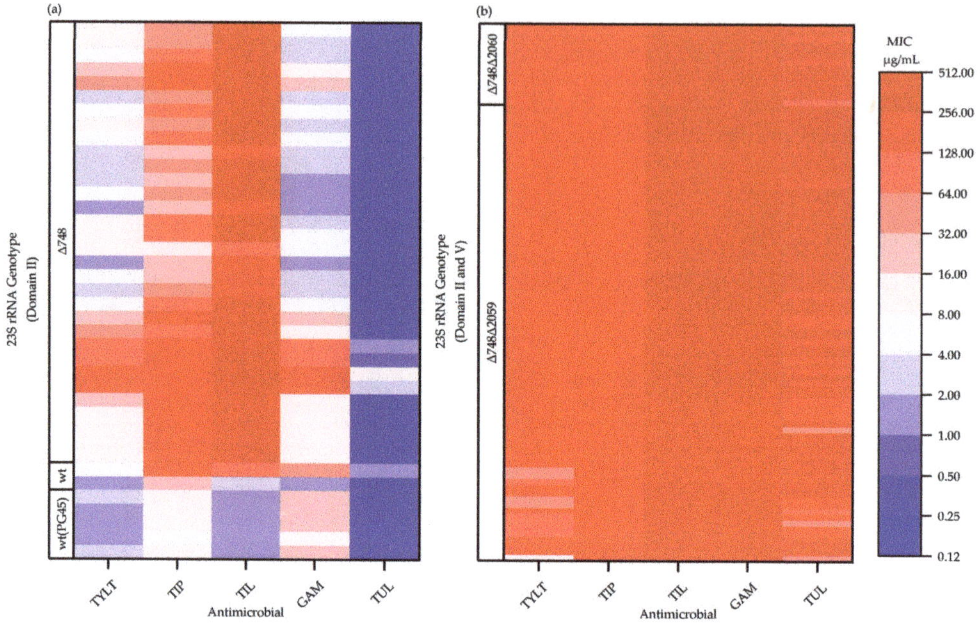

Figure 1. Minimum inhibitory concentrations (MIC) of *Mycoplasma bovis* isolates (n = 126) for tylosin (TYLT), tilmicosin (TIL), tildipirosin (TIP), gamithromycin (GAM), and tulathromycin (TUL), and the corresponding 23S rRNA genotype: (**a**) wildtype (wt) or mutations in domain II only (Δ748); (**b**) mutations in domain II and V (Δ748Δ2059, Δ748Δ2060). The MIC values for the five *M. bovis* PG45 replicates [wt(PG45)] are presented. TYLT, TIL, and TIP have a 16-membered core structure; whereas, GAM and TUL have a 15-membered core structure.

Table 4. Number and proportion of *Mycoplasma bovis* isolates (n = 126) resistant (R) or susceptible (S) by 23S rRNA genotype. The 95% binomial proportion confidence interval (Wilson score) is an interval estimate of the probability of the isolate being resistant if it has a particular 23S rRNA genotype.

		23S rRNA Genotype^{+}			
		Wildtype	**Δ748 only**	**Δ748Δ2059**	**Δ748Δ2060**
TUL	R/S	0/2	0/32	78/0	14/0
	Proportion (95% CI)	0 (0–0.66)	0 (0–0.11)	1 (0.95–1)	1 (0.78–1)
GAM	R/S	1/1	13/19	78/0	14/0
	Proportion (95% CI)	0.50 (0.09–0.91)	0.41 (0.26–0.58)	1 (0.95–1)	1 (0.78–1)
TYLT	R/S	0/2	19/13	78/0	14/0
	Proportion (95% CI)	0 (0–0.66)	0.59 (0.42–0.74)	1 (0.95–1)	1 (0.78–1)
TIL	R/S	1/1	32/0	78/0	14/0
	Proportion (95% CI)	0.50 (0.09–0.91)	1 (0.89–1)	1 (0.95–1)	1 (0.78–1)
TIP	R/S	2/0	32/0	78/0	14/0
	Proportion (95% CI)	1 (0.34–1)	1 (0.89–1)	1 (0.95–1)	1 (0.78–1)
Total		2	32	78	14

GAM—gamithromycin, TIL—tilmicosin, TIP—tildipirosin, TUL—tulathromycin, and TYLT—tylosin. $^{+}$ Positioning of the alleles is based on *Escherichia coli* numbering.

The level of agreement in the classification of resistance between the presence of a mutation in domain V in the 23S rRNA genotype and phenotype (MIC values) varied by macrolide. The kappa correlation coefficient was perfect (1.000) for TUL, moderate (0.676) for GAM, weak (0.536) for TYLT, essentially nonexistent (0.042) for TIL, and could not be determined for TIP because all isolates were resistant regardless of the genotype. Despite these differences, all isolates with a mutation in domain V of the 23S rRNA genotype (Δ748Δ2059 and Δ748Δ2060) were resistant to all macrolides. However, mutations in domain V also occurred in the presence of a mutation in domain II at position 748.

2.4. L4 and L22 Ribosomal Proteins

All isolates had a nonsynonymous mutation Gln93His (*M. bovis* PG45 number; equivalent to Gln90His using *E. coli* numbering) in the L22 ribosomal protein. There were multiple nonsynonymous L4 mutations: Ser18Thr, Thr43Ala, Ala44Thr, Glu50Thr, Ala51Thr, Ala51Ser, Ser55Ala, Thr57Ala, Val69Ala, Ala70Thr, Glu75Ala, Ala86Thr, and Ala101Thr (*M. bovis* PG45 numbering) with three different nonsynonymous mutations at two positions in proximity to the MLS_B binding pocket Gly185Arg, Gly185Ala, Thr186Pro (*M. bovis* PG45 numbering; equivalent to position 64 and 65 using *E. coli* numbering, respectively).

Twelve isolates had a nonsynonymous mutation in the L4 ribosomal protein in residues proximal to the MLS_B binding pocket. Four had two nonsynonymous mutations Gly185Ala and Thr186Pro, and eight had a single nonsynonymous mutation Gly185Arg (Table 5). All isolates had Gln93His mutations in L22 as well. All isolates with the two nonsynonymous mutations (Gly185Ala and Thr186Pro) also had mutations in domain II of the 23S rRNA gene (Δ748). The eight isolates with a single nonsynonymous mutation (Gly185Arg) had various 23S rRNA genotypes: wildtype (n = 1), Δ748 (n = 1), and Δ748Δ2059 (n = 6). Overall, isolates with a Δ748 mutation in the 23S rRNA gene and mutations in L4 and L22 near the MLS_B binding pocket were resistant (MICs ≥16 μg/mL) to GAM, TIL, TIP and TYLT; but susceptible (MICs ≤ 8 μg/mL) to TUL.

Table 5. Presence of ribosomal protein mutations in different 23S genotype groups and corresponding minimum inhibitory concentrations (MIC) values.

23S rRNA Genotype⁺	MIC (μg/mL)					Ribosomal Proteins‡	
	GAM	TIL	TIP	TUL	TYLT	L4	L22
wildtype (PG45)	8–16	1	4–8	0.25	1–2	Gly185, Thr186	Gln93
wildtype	32	64	>128	1	4	Gly185Arg	Gln93His
Δ748	128	>256	>128	2	128	Gly185Ala, Thr186Pro	Gln93His
	128	>256	>128	8	128	Gly185Ala, Thr186Pro	Gln93His
	64	>256	>128	0.5	64	Gly185Ala, Thr186Pro	Gln93His
	64	>256	>128	1	64	Gly185Ala, Thr186Pro	Gln93His
	16	256	128	0.25	32	Gly185Arg	Gln93His
Δ748Δ2059	>256	>256	>128	>256	>128	Gly185Arg	Gln93His
	>256	>256	>128	256	>128	Gly185Arg	Gln93His
	>256	>256	>128	>256	>128	Gly185Arg	Gln93His
	>256	>256	>128	128	64	Gly185Arg	Gln93His
	>256	>256	>128	128	64	Gly185Arg	Gln93His
	>256	>256	>128	32	64	Gly185Arg	Gln93His

⁺ Positioning of the alleles is based on *Escherichia coli* numbering. ‡ Positioning of amino acids is based on *Mycoplasma bovis* PG45 numbering.

3. Discussion

This study was unique in that it assessed the concordance between the genotypes and phenotypes of *M. bovis* for antimicrobial resistance (AMR) to five macrolides used to control and treat bovine respiratory disease in feedlot cattle. Of note was the inclusion of TUL, which is the most commonly used antimicrobial for BRD prophylaxis, but a pharmaceutical that has not been assessed in previous genotype–phenotype AMR studies [13,31,32,47]. This is salient because even though macrolides have a similar antibacterial mode of action, they differ in the size of the macrocyclic lactone ring and associated side-chains [48]. As a result, each macrolide has a slightly different binding affinity for domains II and V of 23S rRNA. Thus, one or more mutations within these domains may lead to very different antimicrobial susceptibility testing (AST) results. Exemplars are TUL, TIL, and TIP, where a single mutation in domain II (Δ748) conferred resistance to TIL and TIP, but not to TUL. This is consistent with the modeling of the *E. coli* ribosome, wherein TUL interacts primarily at A2058 of 23S rRNA, but is too small to span the ribosomal tunnel and interact with G748 in domain II [48]. This finding is of interest because previous genotype studies did not include TUL.

Within the 23S rRNA gene, mutations in domain V occurred at position 2059 or 2060, but not both. In contrast, Lerner et al. [31] identified two isolates with mutations in both *rrl* alleles in domain V, but at different positions (2058 and 2059). Furthermore, others have reported mutations at position 2058 in *M. bovis* [31,47,49], an outcome that was not found in the current study. Isolates with differing alleles at a given position in domain V were resistant to all five macrolides, which is consistent with a previous study in which *Mycoplasma* spp. having a heterozygous mutation in domain V conferred resistance [33]. Additionally, mutations at position 2060 have been reported in *M. bovis* isolates that are resistant to lincomycin [32], an antimicrobial with a mechanism of action similar to macrolides [7,26]. These differences in position, albeit in close proximity to one another, could reflect differences in the selective pressure of specific antimicrobials as a result of differences in use across production systems. Despite these differences, the increased resistance of *M. bovis* to macrolides as a result of mutations in domain II and domain V is consistent with previous reports [13,31,32,47].

Overall, concordance was observed between 23S rRNA genotype and AMR phenotype, which highlights the utility of molecular targets as a viable alternative to in vitro AST. Isolates with combined mutations in domain II and V binding sites of 23S rRNA gene (Δ748Δ2059 and Δ748Δ2060) all demonstrated resistance to TUL, GAM, and TYLT. Whereas regardless of genotype, >99% of all isolates were resistant to TIP and TIL. The accumulation of SNPs in domain II and V of the 23S rRNA gene and the relationship to increasing MIC values, and therefore inferred resistance, has been reported for TYLT and TIL in *M. bovis* by Hata et al. [13]. Lui and Douthwaite [50] also demonstrated that monomethylation at positions G748 and A2058 acted synergistically to increase TYLT resistance. In both the Lerner et al. [31] study and the current study, the existence of mutations in both the II and V domains correlated with MICs for TYLT and TIL that were indicative of clinical resistance. However, it has also been reported that some *M. bovis* isolates with elevated MICs to TYLT and TIL only have a mutation in domain V, without a concurrent mutation at position 748 [31,47], while others had a change at 748 without a mutation in domain V [32].

Given that TIP and TIL are both derivatives of TYLT, the similarities in the level of resistance to these macrolides is not surprising. These three macrolides vary in the groups that decorate C5, C6, and C14 of their shared 16-membered core structure. As high levels of resistance (>99%) to both TIL and TIP was present, it was difficult to correlate phenotype and genotype. However, as per previous reports [9,10,16,17] the very high MIC values for these two antimicrobials indicate that they are unsuitable for treating mycoplasmosis in cattle.

The associations of mutations in the L4 and L22 ribosomal proteins with susceptibility phenotypes were less clear than those of domains II and V of the 23S rRNA gene. Zhao et al. [51] reported that mutations in these ribosomal proteins lead to increased macrolide resistance in *M. pneumonia*. In the current study, mutations in L4 and L22 were associated with elevated MICs for GAM, TYLT, TIP, and TIL. Given that these ribosomal proteins form the narrowest constriction of the protein exit tunnel [52], with both having loops that extend adjacent to macrolide binding sites [53], the presence of mutations is consistent with the AST phenotypes. All isolates (n = 126) also had mutations in L22 relative to the type strain, a result more prevalent than reported by Lerner et al. [31], where the nonsynonymous mutation Gln90His (*E. coli* numbering) in L22 was observed in 75% of isolates. Again, these differences across studies are likely related to increased antimicrobial selection pressure placed on the western Canadian isolates.

There was a very low prevalence of the *M. bovis* type strain PG45 genotype (1.6%) in this study compared to Hata et al. [13], who observed this genotype in 12.3% of 203 bovine isolates from Japan. Lerner et al. [31] found that this genotype in about half of the 54 isolates from cattle originating in the Middle East, Europe, and Australia. Variation in the proportion of wildtype *M. bovis* isolates circulating within cattle populations is undoubtedly related to differences in cattle production systems and antimicrobial use. In western Canada, most beef calves are weaned in the fall of the year and sold at auctions where they are commingled with cohorts from other farms. These newly weaned calves are then transported to feedlots where they are processed on-arrival. In addition to these stressors, these events occur when the weather can be also be inclement. Therefore, calves deemed to be at high-risk of developing BRD are administered macrolides, often TUL, on-arrival. Our data indicate that over time this practice has selected against wildtype genotypes and for the emergence of macrolide resistant genotypes. Significantly, not only has macrolide resistance in western Canadian feedlot cattle been increasing, it is also not uncommon to recover macrolide resistant *M. bovis* isolates from the nasopharynx of healthy cattle at feedlot arrival [11]. While feedlots could rotate macrolides with tetracyclines or florfenicol, as a strategy to reduce resistance, this practice requires timely AST data or otherwise it may exacerbate antimicrobial resistance.

The study had a number of potential weaknesses. The wildtype 23S rRNA genotype essentially served as a control group; however, there were only two isolates in this group. This was unfortunate since one of two wildtype isolates were resistant to GAM and TIL, and both resistant to TIP. Additionally, control testing of healthy animals was not performed at the time of sampling diseased or dead animals. However, this study was not intended as a survey of macrolide susceptibility, but rather an investigation of the relationship between genotype and phenotype. Therefore, the healthy animals were sampled with the intent of culturing phenotypically susceptible isolates to serve as a basis of comparison to the abundance of resistant isolates derived from dead cattle. The other weaknesses were that the isolates were not uniformly spread over all 12 production years, and most isolates came from dead animals that had received extensive antimicrobial therapy prior to death. The study, however, also had some notable strengths. The relatively large number of isolates came from cattle that were sourced from a broad geographic area; samples were collected over 12 production years; from multiple anatomical locations; and from healthy, diseased and dead cattle.

Conventional antimicrobial susceptibility testing for *M. bovis* is time-consuming and technically demanding, making it unsuitable for monitoring antimicrobial resistance in real-time within a feedlot. This is an issue because prudent use guidelines for antimicrobial use are predicated on AST. This study, and others, have shown a clear linkage between genotypes and macrolide resistance, providing an avenue for developing a rapid, accurate, and cost-effective molecular based test for *M. bovis*, similar to what has been done for *Mycoplasma genitalium* [34,54,55]. This test could be used to assess *M. bovis* isolates obtained from nasapharyngeal swabs, or for conducting pen-level AST surveillance by testing isolates found in shared watering bowls.

4. Materials and Methods

4.1. Animals and Sample Collection

Mycoplasma bovis isolates were cultured from a cross-section of clinical samples derived from different anatomical regions (nasopharynx, lung, and joint) of western Canadian feedlot cattle over 12 production years (2006–2018). Deep nasopharyngeal swabs from live cattle were taken in accordance with Animal Use Protocols (#20070023; #20170021) approved by the University of Saskatchewan's Animal Research Ethics Board and Lethbridge Research Center's Animal Care Committee (#1641).

Sampling was performed as described in Jelinski et al. [11]. Briefly, doubled-guarded uterine swabs (Reproduction Resources, Walworth, WI, USA) were used to obtain deep nasopharyngeal (DNP) samples from healthy and diseased cattle. The diseased cattle were identified by feedlot personnel trained in recognizing the clinical signs of BRD (dyspnea, depression, nasal discharge, anorexia, and fever). Swabs were immediately placed in Ames media (Mai, Ames Media, Product 49203, Spring Valley, WI, USA).

All other swabs or tissues were collected from animals purposively sampled by feedlot veterinarians recruited to provide clinical case material for the study. Samples were obtained by the veterinarians from animals that on postmortem examination were found to have pathological lesions consistent with *M. bovis* pneumonia or chronic pneumonia and polyarthritis syndrome (CPPS). Specifically, the lungs had gross pathology consistent with caseonecrotic pneumonia and/or chronic bronchopneumonia. A minimum 3 × 3 cm lung sample was excised and if septic arthritis was concurrently observed, then the diseased joints were sampled by swabbing, aspirating synovial fluid, or excising synovial tissue.

Tissue and fluid specimens were stored at −20 °C, and batch shipped by courier. Upon receipt, samples were stored at −80 °C until culturing. For each sample, the following metadata were recorded: date of sampling, type of sample (swab, tissue, joint fluid), anatomical location (nasopharynx, lung, joint), and disease status (healthy, diseased, dead).

4.2. *Mycoplasma Culture and Isolation*

Selective culture was performed on the DNP swabs and on swabs of the cut tissue surfaces as previously described by Jelinski et al. [11]. Due to the extended time span of sample collection, there were slight differences in isolation methods and media over the course of the study. Samples collected between 2006 to 2008 were cultured using Hayflick's media (made in-house), whereas in subsequent years samples were cultured using pleuropneumonia-like organism (PPLO) broth and agar (BD Difco, Fisher Scientific, Waltham, MA, USA), supplemented with 10 g/L yeast extract (BD Diagnostic Systems, Fisher Scientific, Waltham, MA, USA), and 20% horse serum (Invitrogen, Fisher Scientific) [11,56]. Where specified, the media was supplemented with 0.05% thallium (I) acetate, 500 U/mL penicillin G, and/or 0.5% sodium pyruvate (Sigma-Aldrich, St. Louis, MO, USA).

Cultures derived from samples were filtered through 0.45 and 0.20 μm filters (Basix, VWR International, Radnor, PA, USA), and were used to inoculate PPLO broth with 0.05% thallium (I) acetate, 500 U/mL penicillin G, and 0.5% sodium pyruvate, and grown in a 5% CO_2 atmosphere with 75% humidity at 37 °C. Cultures with visible growth were streaked onto PPLO agar with 0.05% thallium (I) acetate and 500 U/mL penicillin G and incubated for 3–6 days. An isolated colony with characteristic "fried-egg" morphology was picked, replated on PPLO agar, and incubated for 72 h. Up to three individual colonies per sample were used to inoculate separate aliquots of PPLO broth with 0.05% thallium (I) acetate and 500 U/mL penicillin G. After 48 h of growth, each culture was separately stored in PPLO with glycerol (20%, *v*/*v*) at −80 °C. From the three possible cultures, a single culture was chosen to inoculate PPLO media for DNA extraction and antimicrobial susceptibility testing.

4.3. *DNA Extraction and Identification*

Mycoplasma bovis isolates were grown in PPLO media for 48 h and the genomic DNA was extracted using the GenElute Bacterial Genomic DNA Kit (Sigma-Aldrich, St. Louis, MO, USA). The DNA was extracted following manufacturer's instructions for Gram negative bacteria with the final elution buffer replaced with 10 mM Tris (pH 8.5). Extracted genomic DNA was assessed for quality using gel electrophoresis and quantified fluorometrically using Qubit (thermo Fisher Scientific, Waltham, MA, USA). Cultures were confirmed as *M. bovis*, based on confirmation of the presence of *uvr*C [57] and sequencing of the 16S rRNA gene [58]. The 16S rRNA amplicon was purified using a QIAquick PCR purification kit (Qiagen, Nevlo, Netherlands) and sent to Macrogen (Seoul, South Korea) for Sanger sequencing with the amplification primers. Forward and reverse sequences were assembled and edited using the Staden Package (version 1.6-r, http://staden.sourceforge.net/). The resulting sequences were compared to the National Center for Biotechnology Information (NCBI) nonredundant nucleotide database (nr) using BLASTn.

4.4. *Whole Genome Sequencing and Assembly*

Genomic DNA was prepared for sequencing using Illumina Nextera XT DNA Library Preparation (Illumina Inc., San Diego, CA, USA) and sequenced on a Illumina MiSeq platform using the MiSeq v2 Reagent Kit to generate 250 bp paired-end reads. Illumina reads were trimmed using Trimmomatic v0.38 [59] with settings slidingwindow:5:15 leading:5 trailing:5 and minlen:50. Genomes were assembled with *M. bovis* PG45 as the reference genome (CP002188) using BWA-MEM v0.7.10-r789 [60] with default settings, producing SAM formatted assemblies. SAMtools [61] was used to convert the assemblies to BAM files and then sort and index for further processing. The Picard v2.18.4-SNAPSHOT [62] marked and removed duplicate reads from the BAM file. The Genome Analysis ToolKit v3.4-46-gbc02625 was used to perform local indel realignment and base quality score recalibration to improve the alignment quality, according to GATK best practices pipeline [63]. Consensus sequences for each assembly were created from each BAM file using bcftools [61]. This was performed by piping results from bcftools mpileup to bcftools call to create a vcf file for each BAM file. Each vcf file was used as input for vcfutils vcf2fq to generate a consensus fastq file. The fastq files were converted to fasta files using a bash script.

Genes encoding for 23S rRNA (*rrl3* and *rrl4*), L4 (*rplD*), and L22 (*rplV*) ribosomal proteins were identified using BLASTn [64] to compare *M. bovis* strain PG45 genes to the assembled genomes. For *rrl3* and *rrl4*, the closest matching sequence to the start of the genome being analyzed was identified as *rrl3*, the furthest as *rrl4*. As two start sites have been proposed for ribosomal protein L4, for the purposes of this study the position of *rplD* and overall numbering was based on locus ID MBOVPG45_0263. Extraction of gene sequences was performed using the start and ends of the match as reported by BLASTn for input to SAMtools faidx [61]. Genes of interest extracted from each isolate were aligned with the equivalent region in the *M. bovis* PG45 reference genome (CP002188.1) in Geneious Prime 2020.0.5 (https://www.geneious.com) using MUSCLE to identify SNPs with a minimum variant frequency of 0.01. For L4 and L22 ribosomal protein gene alignments, they were translated using the *Mycoplasma* spp. genetic code. To verify the nucleotide composition in *rrl3* and *rrl4* at positions within hairpin 35 in domain II and the peptidyl transferase loop in domain V within the MLS_B binding pocket [65], the SAM files were queried for ambiguity to determine the representative nucleotide(s). In cases of ambiguity, the percent of reads for a given allele was >20%. The raw paired reads for the isolates used in this study are available at NCBI SRA (www.ncbi.nlm.nih.gov/sra) with BioProject ID PRJNA642970.

The *M. bovis* sequences were aligned to their respective 23S rRNA (*rrlA*), L4 (*rplD*), or L22 ribosomal protein (*rplV*) genes isolated from the *E. coli* K12 substrain MG1655 genome to determine equivalent positioning to generate numbering to allow for comparison between different studies and bacterial species.

4.5. Antimicrobial Susceptibility Testing

Antimicrobial susceptibility (AST) was determined using a microdilution assay, in a Sensititre™ (Trek Diagnostics, Oakwood, GA, USA) plate format and a customized panel designed to assess the antimicrobials most commonly used in North American feedlots for the treatment and control of BRD. The panel consisted of ten antimicrobials as described by Jelinski et al. [11], five of which were macrolides: tildipirosin (TIP; 0.12–128 μg/mL), gamithromycin (GAM; 0.25–256 μg/mL), tulathromycin (TUL; 0.25–256 μg/mL), tilmicosin (TIL; 1–256 μg/mL), and tylosin tartrate (TYLT; 1–128 μg/mL). AlamarBlue (thermoFisher Scientific, DAL1100), a color redox indicator, was used to assess growth in each well based on a blue to pink color transition.

The AST procedure began by inoculating an *M. bovis* isolate previously stored at −80 °C in 20% glycerol into PPLO broth with 0.5% pyruvate and incubating for 72 h at 5% CO_2 with 75% humidity at 37 °C. Broth cultures were then subcultured into neat PPLO (without antibiotics) and incubated for 24 h. Following incubation, the optical density (OD) at 450 nm was determined using a NanoDrop One Spectrophotometer (Fisher Scientific, Waltham, MA, USA) and the culture adjusted to an $OD_{450} = 0.1$. The adjusted culture was diluted up to 100×, and 120 μL of the diluted culture used to inoculate 6 mL of PPLO in 2× alamarBlue. Each well of a Sensititre™ plate was inoculated to a final concentration of 10^3 to 5×10^5 CFU/mL with 50 μL of culture in 2× alamarBlue in 50 μL of media with each of antimicrobials within a series of Sensititre wells (final working concentration of alamarBlue: 1×; final well volume:

100 μL). Plates were sealed with a CO_2 permeable film, and incubated for 48–72 h. Minimum inhibitory concentrations (MICs) were determined by visual assessment of plates at 48 and 72 h, based on a blue to pink colour change. The *M. bovis* reference strain (*Mycoplasma bovis* ATCC® 25523™) was tested five times for quality control.

4.6. Clinical Breakpoints

As there are no established macrolide breakpoints for *M. bovis,* they were extrapolated from other members of the bacterial BRD complex (i.e., *Mannheimia haemolytica, Pasteurella multocida, Histophilus somni*) and human *Mycoplasma* spp., as described previously in Jelinski et al. [11]. The resistance breakpoints were ≥8 μg/mL for TIP, GAM, TIL, and TYLT, and ≥32 μg/mL for TUL.

4.7. Statistical Analysis

As *rrl3* and *rrl4* genes in the reference sequence for *M. bovis* PG45 differ by only a single nucleotide, alleles in each isolate could not be assigned to a specific locus. Instead, allele(s) at a given position were reported and isolates were grouped into genotypes according to the presence of mutation(s) in domain II and V. This created four 23S rRNA genotype groups: wildtype, Δ748 only, Δ748Δ2059, and Δ748Δ2060.

As phenotypically resistant and susceptible isolates were derived from cattle in each health status cohort (healthy, diseased, and dead), all isolates were analyzed together regardless of their source. Confidence intervals were calculated using the Wilson score interval method for estimating intervals for proportions. The confidence intervals were used to represent the antimicrobial resistance for a given 23S rRNA genotype using Epitools [66]. To assess the agreement in classification of resistance between the presence of a mutation in domain V of the 23S rRNA genotype and phenotype (MIC value), the Cohen's kappa statistic interpretation criteria (value, level of agreement): 0–0.20, none; 0.21–0.39, minimal; 0.40–0.59, weak; 0.60–0.79, moderate; 0.80–0.90, strong; >0.90, almost perfect [67] were calculated using a commercial statistical program (SPSS 26, IBM SPSS Statistics version 26, IBM Corporation, Armonk, NY, USA). All descriptive statistics were calculated using a commercial spreadsheet software (Microsoft Excel version 15; Microsoft Corporation, Redmond, Washington, WA, USA).

5. Conclusions

Given that antimicrobials are the primary preventative and therapeutic tool to combat *M. bovis* infections in feedlot cattle, ongoing assessment of antimicrobial susceptibility remains crucial to maintaining the utility of these drugs and facilitating antimicrobial stewardship practices. However, the comparatively slow growth of *M. bovis* yields longer turn-around times when exclusively using culture-based methods of assessment, which can impede timely decision making on antimicrobial use. In our study, we were able to identify mutations in domains II and V of the 23S rRNA genes that are associated with increased resistance to macrolides which show a clear linkage between genotype and phenotypic macrolide resistance (AST). These findings add strong support for utilizing rapid, accurate, and cost-effective molecular based tests for assessing the susceptibility of *M. bovis* to macrolides.

Author Contributions: Conceptualization, M.D.J., T.A.M.; Methodology, M.D.J., T.A.M., A.K., M.W., R.Z, S.A.-L., J.E.H., A.C.R.; Formal Analysis, A.K., M.W., R.Z., S.P.; Investigation, M.D.J., A.K., R.Z.; Resources, M.D.J., T.A.M., J.E.H.; Data Curation, M.D.J., A.K., M.W.; Writing—Original Draft Preparation, A.K., M.DJ., T.A.M.; Writing—Review and Editing, A.K., M.J., T.A.M., M.W., R.Z., S.A.-L., S.P., J.E.H., A.C.R.; Supervision, M.D.J., T.A.M., J.E.H. Funding Acquisition, M.D.J., T.A.M. All authors have read and agreed to the published version of the manuscript.

Funding: Funding for this study was provided by the Saskatchewan Agricultural Development Fund (Grants #20060116, #20130170, #20160253) and the Canadian Cattlemen's Association, Beef Cattle Research Council Division (Grant ANH.30.17).

Acknowledgments: the authors would like to express their appreciation to: Karen Register, Research Microbiologist, USDA, Ames, IA and Manual Chirino-Trejo, Professor Emeritus, Western College of Veterinary Medicine, for their assistance and guidance in the processing of the samples. They also thank Karen Gesy

(University of Saskatchewan), Champika Fernando (University of Saskatchewan), and Rodrigo Ortega-Polo (Lethbridge Research and Development Centre) for their assistance in culturing, sequencing, and bioinformatics, respectively. We also wish to acknowledge and thank the veterinary practices that collected samples and the feedlot producers for allowing their cattle to be sampled.

Conflicts of Interest: the authors declare no conflict of interest.

References

1. Nicholas, R.A.J.; Ayling, R.D. Mycoplasma bovis: Disease, diagnosis, and control. *Res. Vet. Sci.* **2003**, *74*, 105–112. [CrossRef]
2. Maunsell, F.P.; Woolums, A.R.; Francoz, D.; Rosenbusch, R.F.; Step, D.L.; Wilson, D.J.; Janzen, E.D. Mycoplasma bovis infections in cattle. *J. Vet. Intern. Med.* **2011**, *25*, 772–783. [CrossRef]
3. Gagea, M.I.; Bateman, K.G.; Shanahan, R.A.; van Dreumel, T.; McEwen, B.J.; Carman, S.; Archambault, M.; Caswell, J.L. Naturally Occurring Mycoplasma Bovis—Associated Pneumonia and Polyarthritis in Feedlot Beef Calves. *J. Vet. Diagn. Investig.* **2006**, *18*, 29–40. [CrossRef]
4. Caswell, J.L.; Bateman, K.G.; Cai, H.Y.; Castillo-Alcala, F. Mycoplasma bovis in Respiratory Disease of Feedlot Cattle. *Vet. Clin. N. Am. Food Anim.* **2010**, *26*, 365–379. [CrossRef]
5. Krysak, D.E. Chronic pneumonia and polyarthritis syndrome in a feedlot calf. *Can. Vet. J.* **2006**, *47*, 1019–1022.
6. Caswell, J.L.; Archambault, M. Mycoplasma bovis pneumonia in cattle. *Anim. Health Res. Rev.* **2007**, *8*, 161–186. [CrossRef]
7. Lysnyansky, I.; Ayling, R.D. Mycoplasma bovis: Mechanisms of Resistance and Trends in Antimicrobial Susceptibility. *Front. Microbiol.* **2016**, *7*, 595. [CrossRef] [PubMed]
8. Hendrick, S.H.; Bateman, K.G.; Rosengren, L.B. The effect of antimicrobial treatment and preventive strategies on bovine respiratory disease and genetic relatedness and antimicrobial resistance of Mycoplasma bovis isolates in a western Canadian feedlot. *Can. Vet. J.* **2013**, *54*, 1146–1156. [PubMed]
9. Anholt, R.M.; Klima, C.; Allan, N.; Matheson-Bird, H.; Schatz, C.; Ajitkumar, P.; Otto, S.J.; Peters, D.; Schmid, K.; Olson, M.; et al. Antimicrobial Susceptibility of Bacteria That Cause Bovine Respiratory Disease Complex in Alberta, Canada. *Front. Vet. Sci.* **2017**, *4*, 207. [CrossRef] [PubMed]
10. Cai, H.Y.; McDowall, R.; Parker, L.; Kaufman, E.I.; Caswell, J.L. Changes in antimicrobial susceptibility profiles of Mycoplasma bovis over time. *Can. J. Vet. Res.* **2019**, *83*, 34–41. [PubMed]
11. Jelinski, M.; Kinnear, A.; Gesy, K.; Andrés-Lasheras, S.; Zaheer, R.; Weese, S.; McAllister, T.A. Antimicrobial Sensitivity Testing of Mycoplasma bovis Isolates Derived from Western Canadian Feedlot Cattle. *Microorganisms* **2020**, *8*, 124. [CrossRef] [PubMed]
12. Rosenbusch, R.F.; Kinyon, J.M.; Apley, M.; Funk, N.D.; Smith, S.; Hoffman, L.J. In Vitro Antimicrobial Inhibition Profiles of Mycoplasma Bovis Isolates Recovered from Various Regions of the United States from 2002 to 2003. *J. Vet. Diagn. Investig.* **2005**, *17*, 436–441. [CrossRef]
13. Hata, E.; Harada, T.; Itoh, M. Relationship between Antimicrobial Susceptibility and Multilocus Sequence Type of Mycoplasma bovis Isolates and Development of a Method for Rapid Detection of Point Mutations Involved in Decreased Susceptibility to Macrolides, Lincosamides, Tetracyclines, and Spectinomycin. *Appl. Environ. Microbiol.* **2019**, *85*, e00575-19. [CrossRef] [PubMed]
14. Ayling, R.D.; Baker, S.E.; Nicholas, R.A.J.; Peek, M.L.; Simon, A.J. Comparison of in vitro activity of danofloxacin, florfenicol, oxytetracycline, spectinomycin and tilmicosin against recent field isolates of Mycoplasma bovis. *Vet. Rec.* **2000**, *146*, 745–747. [CrossRef] [PubMed]
15. Gerchman, I.; Levisohn, S.; Mikula, I.; Lysnyansky, I. In vitro antimicrobial susceptibility of Mycoplasma bovis isolated in Israel from local and imported cattle. *Vet. Microbiol.* **2009**, *137*, 268–275. [CrossRef] [PubMed]
16. Gautier-Bouchardon, A.V.; Ferré, S.; Le Grand, D.; Paoli, A.; Gay, E.; Poumarat, F. Overall decrease in the susceptibility of Mycoplasma bovis to antimicrobials over the past 30 years in France. *PLoS ONE* **2014**, *9*, e87672. [CrossRef]
17. Sulyok, K.M.; Kreizinger, Z.; Fekete, L.; Hrivnák, V.; Magyar, T.; Jánosi, S.; Schweitzer, N.; Turcsányi, I.; Makrai, L.; Erdélyi, K.; et al. Antibiotic susceptibility profiles of Mycoplasma bovis strains isolated from cattle in Hungary, Central Europe. *BMC Vet. Res.* **2014**, *10*, 256. [CrossRef]

18. Heuvelink, A.; Reugebrink, C.; Mars, J. Antimicrobial susceptibility of Mycoplasma bovis isolates from veal calves and dairy cattle in the Netherlands. *Vet. Microbiol.* **2016**, *189*, 1–7. [CrossRef]
19. Klein, U.; de Jong, A.; Moyaert, H.; El Garch, F.; Leon, R.; Richard-Mazet, A.; Rose, M.; Maes, D.; Pridmore, A.; Thomson, J.R.; et al. Antimicrobial susceptibility monitoring of Mycoplasma hyopneumoniae and Mycoplasma bovis isolated in Europe. *Vet. Microbiol.* **2017**, *204*, 188–193. [CrossRef]
20. Mzyk, D.A.; Bublitz, C.M.; Martinez, M.N.; Davis, J.L.; Baynes, R.E.; Smith, G.W. Impact of bovine respiratory disease on the pharmacokinetics of danofloxacin and tulathromycin in different ages of calves. *PLoS ONE* **2019**, *14*, e0218864. [CrossRef]
21. Griffin, D. Economic Impact Associated with Respiratory Disease in Beef Cattle. *Vet. Clin. N. Am. Large Anim. Pract.* **1997**, *13*, 367–377. [CrossRef]
22. Nickell, J.S.; White, B.J. Metaphylactic Antimicrobial therapy for Bovine Respiratory Disease in Stocker and Feedlot Cattle. *Vet. Clin. N. Am. Food Anim.* **2010**, *26*, 285–301. [CrossRef] [PubMed]
23. Brault, S.A.; Hannon, S.J.; Gow, S.P.; Warr, B.N.; Withell, J.; Song, J.; Williams, C.M.; Otto, S.J.G.; Booker, C.W.; Morley, P.S. Antimicrobial Use on 36 Beef Feedlots in Western Canada: 2008–2012. *Front. Vet. Sci.* **2019**, *6*, 329. [CrossRef] [PubMed]
24. Owen, J.R.; Noyes, N.; Young, A.E.; Prince, D.J.; Blanchard, P.C.; Lehenbauer, T.W.; Aly, S.S.; Davis, J.H.; O'Rourke, S.M.; Abdo, Z.; et al. Whole-Genome Sequencing and Concordance Between Antimicrobial Susceptibility Genotypes and Phenotypes of Bacterial Isolates Associated with Bovine Respiratory Disease. *G3 Genes Genomes Genet.* **2017**, *7*, 3059–3071. [CrossRef] [PubMed]
25. Calcutt, M.J.; Lysnyansky, I.; Sachse, K.; Fox, L.K.; Nicholas, R.A.J.; Ayling, R.D. Gap analysis of Mycoplasma bovis disease, diagnosis and control: An aid to identify future development requirements. *Transbound. Emerg. Dis.* **2018**, *65*, 91–109. [CrossRef]
26. Zaheer, R.; Cook, S.R.; Klima, C.L.; Stanford, K.; Alexander, T.; Topp, E.; Read, R.R.; McAllister, T.A. Effect of subtherapeutic vs. Therapeutic administration of macrolides on antimicrobial resistance in Mannheimia haemolytica and enterococci isolated from beef cattle. *Front. Microbiol.* **2013**, *4*, 133. [CrossRef]
27. Hansen, L.H.; Mauvais, P.; Douthwaite, S. The macrolide–ketolide antibiotic binding site is formed by structures in domains II and V of 23S ribosomal RNA. *Mol. Microbiol.* **1999**, *31*, 623–631. [CrossRef]
28. Moore, P.B.; Steitz, T.A. The Structural Basis of Large Ribosomal Subunit Function. *Annu. Rev. Biochem.* **2003**, *72*, 813–850. [CrossRef]
29. Dinos, G.P. The macrolide antibiotic renaissance. *Br. J. Pharmacol.* **2017**, *174*, 2967–2983. [CrossRef]
30. Demczuk, W.; Martin, I.; Peterson, S.; Bharat, A.; Van Domselaar, G.; Graham, M.; Lefebvre, B.; Allen, V.; Hoang, L.; Tyrrell, G.; et al. Genomic Epidemiology and Molecular Resistance Mechanisms of Azithromycin-Resistant Neisseria gonorrhoeae in Canada from 1997 to 2014. *J. Clin. Microbiol.* **2016**, *54*, 1304–1313. [CrossRef]
31. Lerner, U.; Amram, E.; Ayling, R.D.; Mikula, I.; Gerchman, I.; Harrus, S.; Teff, D.; Yogev, D.; Lysnyansky, I. Acquired resistance to the 16-membered macrolides tylosin and tilmicosin by Mycoplasma bovis. *Vet. Microbiol.* **2014**, *168*, 365–371. [CrossRef] [PubMed]
32. Sulyok, K.M.; Kreizinger, Z.; Wehmann, E.; Lysnyansky, I.; Bányai, K.; Marton, S.; Jerzsele, Á.; Rónai, Z.; Turcsányi, I.; Makrai, L.; et al. Mutations Associated with Decreased Susceptibility to Seven Antimicrobial Families in Field and Laboratory-Derived Mycoplasma bovis Strains. *Antimicrob. Agents Chemother.* **2017**, *61*, e01983-16. [CrossRef] [PubMed]
33. Pereyre, S.; Gonzalez, P.; de Barbeyrac, B.; Darnige, A.; Renaudin, H.; Charron, A.; Raherison, S.; Bébéar, C.; Bébéar, C.M. Mutations in 23S rRNA Account for Intrinsic Resistance to Macrolides in Mycoplasma hominis and Mycoplasma fermentans and for Acquired Resistance to Macrolides in M. hominis. *Antimicrob. Agents Chemother.* **2002**, *46*, 3142–3150. [CrossRef] [PubMed]
34. Chrisment, D.; Charron, A.; Cazanave, C.; Pereyre, S.; Bebear, C. Detection of macrolide resistance in Mycoplasma genitalium in France. *J. Antimicrob. Chemother.* **2012**, *67*, 2598–2601. [CrossRef] [PubMed]
35. Canu, A.; Malbruny, B.; Coquemont, M.; Davies, T.A.; Appelbaum, P.C.; Leclercq, R. Diversity of Ribosomal Mutations Conferring Resistance to Macrolides, Clindamycin, Streptogramin, and Telithromycin in Streptococcus pneumoniae. *Antimicrob. Agents Chemother.* **2002**, *46*, 125–131. [CrossRef]
36. Jalava, J.; Vaara, M.; Huovinen, P. Mutation at the position 2058 of the 23S rRNA as a cause of macrolide resistance in Streptococcus pyogenes. *Ann. Clin. Microbiol. Antimicrob.* **2004**, *3*, 5. [CrossRef]

37. Karlsson, E.; Golovliov, I.; Lärkeryd, A.; Granberg, M.; Larsson, E.; Öhrman, C.; Niemcewicz, M.; Birdsell, D.; Wagner, D.M.; Forsman, M.; et al. Clonality of erythromycin resistance in Francisella tularensis. *J. Antimicrob. Chemother.* **2016**, *71*, 2815–2823. [CrossRef]
38. Zaman, S.; Fitzpatrick, M.; Lindahl, L.; Zengel, J. Novel mutations in ribosomal proteins L4 and L22 that confer erythromycin resistance in Escherichia coli. *Mol. Microbiol.* **2007**, *66*, 1039–1050. [CrossRef]
39. Zhu, H.; Wang, H.-P.; Jiang, Y.; Hou, S.-P.; Liu, Y.-J.; Liu, Q.-Z. Mutations in 23S rRNA and ribosomal protein L4 account for resistance in Chlamydia trachomatis strains selected in vitro by macrolide passage. *Andrologia* **2010**, *42*, 274–280. [CrossRef]
40. Peric, M.; Bozdogan, B.; Jacobs, M.R.; Appelbaum, P.C. Effects of an Efflux Mechanism and Ribosomal Mutations on Macrolide Susceptibility of Haemophilus influenzae Clinical Isolates. *Antimicrob. Agents Chemother.* **2003**, *47*, 1017–1022. [CrossRef]
41. CLSI. *Methods for Antimicrobial Susceptibility Testing for Human Mycoplasmas*; Approved Guideline; CLSI Document M43-A; Clinical and Laboratory Standards Institute: Wayne, PA, USA, 2011.
42. CLSI. *Performance Standards for Antimicrobial Disk and Dilution Susceptibility Tests for Bacteria Isolated from Animals*, 4th ed.; CLSI Supplement VET08; Clinical and Laboratory Standards Institute: Wayne, PA, USA, 2018.
43. Gautier-Bouchardon, A.V. Antimicrobial resistance in mycoplasma spp. *Microbiol. Spectrum.* **2018**, *6*, 425–446. [CrossRef]
44. Rottem, S. Interaction of Mycoplasmas with Host Cells. *Physiol. Rev.* **2003**, *83*, 417–432. [CrossRef] [PubMed]
45. Sulyok, K.M.; Bekő, K.; Kreizinger, Z.; Wehmann, E.; Jerzsele, Á.; Rónai, Z.; Turcsányi, I.; Makrai, L.; Szeredi, L.; Jánosi, S.; et al. Development of molecular methods for the rapid detection of antibiotic susceptibility of Mycoplasma bovis. *Vet. Microbiol.* **2018**, *213*, 47–57. [CrossRef] [PubMed]
46. Wise, K.S.; Calcutt, M.J.; Foecking, M.F.; Röske, K.; Madupu, R.; Methé, B.A. Complete Genome Sequence of Mycoplasma bovis Type Strain PG45 (ATCC 25523). *Infect. Immun.* **2011**, *79*, 982–983. [CrossRef]
47. Khalil, D.; Becker, C.A.M.; Tardy, F. Monitoring the Decrease in Susceptibility to Ribosomal RNAs Targeting Antimicrobials and Its Molecular Basis in Clinical Mycoplasma bovis Isolates over Time. *Microb. Drug Resist.* **2017**, *23*, 799–811. [CrossRef]
48. Andersen, N.M.; Poehlsgaard, J.; Warrass, R.; Douthwaite, S. Inhibition of Protein Synthesis on the Ribosome by Tildipirosin Compared with Other Veterinary Macrolides. *Antimicrob. Agents Chemother.* **2012**, *56*, 6033–6036. [CrossRef]
49. Kong, L.C.; Gao, D.; Jia, B.Y.; Wang, Z.; Gao, Y.H.; Pei, Z.H.; Liu, S.M.; Xin, J.Q.; Ma, H.X. Antimicrobial susceptibility and molecular characterization of macrolide resistance of Mycoplasma bovis isolates from multiple provinces in China. *J. Vet. Med. Sci.* **2016**, *78*, 293–296. [CrossRef]
50. Liu, M.; Douthwaite, S. Resistance to the macrolide antibiotic tylosin is conferred by single methylations at 23S rRNA nucleotides G748 and A2058 acting in synergy. *Proc. Natl. Acad. Sci. USA* **2002**, *99*, 14658–14663. [CrossRef]
51. Zhao, F.; Liu, J.; Shi, W.; Huang, F.; Liu, L.; Zhao, S.; Zhang, J. Antimicrobial susceptibility and genotyping of Mycoplasma pneumoniae isolates in Beijing, China, from 2014 to 2016. *Antimicrob. Resist. Infect. Control* **2019**, *8*, 18. [CrossRef]
52. Auerbach-Nevo, T.; Baram, D.; Bashan, A.; Belousoff, M.; Breiner, E.; Davidovich, C.; Cimicata, G.; Eyal, Z.; Halfon, Y.; Krupkin, M.; et al. Ribosomal Antibiotics: Contemporary Challenges. *Antibiotics* **2016**, *5*, 24. [CrossRef]
53. Diner, E.J.; Hayes, C.S. Recombineering Reveals a Diverse Collection of Ribosomal Proteins L4 and L22 that Confer Resistance to Macrolide Antibiotics. *J. Mol. Biol.* **2009**, *386*, 300–315. [CrossRef] [PubMed]
54. Pitt, R.; Fifer, H.; Woodford, N.; Alexander, S. Detection of markers predictive of macrolide and fluoroquinolone resistance in Mycoplasma genitalium from patients attending sexual health services in England. *Sex. Transm. Infect.* **2018**, *94*, 9–13. [CrossRef] [PubMed]
55. Day, M.; Cole, M.; Patel, H.; Fifer, H.; Woodford, N.; Pitt, R. P616 Predictive macrolide and fluoroquinolone resistance markers in mycoplasma genitalium from the UK and ireland. *Sex. Transm. Infect.* **2019**, *95*, A272. [CrossRef]
56. Register, K.B.; Thole, L.; Rosenbush, R.F.; Minion, F.C. Multilocus sequence typing of Mycoplasma bovis reveals host-specific genotypes in cattle versus bison. *Vet. Microbiol.* **2015**, *175*, 92–98. [CrossRef] [PubMed]

57. Register, K.B.; Boatwright, W.D.; Gesy, K.M.; Thacker, T.C.; Jelinski, M.D. Mistaken identity of an open reading frame proposed for PCR-based identification of Mycoplasma bovis and the effect of polymorphisms and insertions on assay performance. *J. Vet. Diagn. Investig.* **2018**, *30*, 637–641. [CrossRef] [PubMed]
58. Miles, K.; McAuliffe, L.; Ayling, R.D.; Nicholas, R.A.J. Rapid detection of Mycoplasma dispar and M. bovirhinis using allele specific polymerase chain reaction protocols. *FEMS Microbiol. Lett.* **2004**, *241*, 103–107. [CrossRef]
59. Bolger, A.M.; Lohse, M.; Usadel, B. Trimmomatic: A flexible trimmer for Illumina sequence data. *Bioinformatics* **2014**, *30*, 2114–2120. [CrossRef]
60. Li, H.; Durbin, R. Fast and accurate short read alignment with Burrows–Wheeler transform. *Bioinformatics* **2009**, *25*, 1754–1760. [CrossRef]
61. Li, H.; Handsaker, B.; Wysoker, A.; Fennell, T.; Ruan, J.; Homer, N.; Marth, G.; Abecasis, G.; Durbin, R. The Sequence Alignment/Map format and SAMtools. *Bioinformatics* **2009**, *25*, 2078–2079. [CrossRef] [PubMed]
62. Broad Institute; GitHub Repository. Picard Toolkit. Available online: http://broadinstitute.github.io/picard/ (accessed on 15 June 2020).
63. Van de Auwera, G.A.; Carneiro, M.O.; Hartl, C.; Poplin, R.; del Angel, G.; Levy-Moonshine, A.; Jordan, T.; Shakir, K.; Roazen, D.; Thibault, J.; et al. From FastQ Data to High-Confidence Variant Calls: The Genome Analysis Toolkit Best Practices Pipeline. *Curr. Protoc. Bioinf.* **2013**, *43*, 11. [CrossRef]
64. Camacho, C.; Coulouris, G.; Avagyan, V.; Ma, N.; Papadopoulos, J.; Bealer, K.; Madden, T.L. BLAST+: Architecture and applications. *BMC Bioinf.* **2009**, *10*, 421. [CrossRef] [PubMed]
65. Vester, B.; Douthwaite, S. Macrolide Resistance Conferred by Base Substitutions in 23S rRNA. *Antimicrob. Agents Chemother.* **2001**, *45*, 1–12. [CrossRef] [PubMed]
66. Sergeant; ESG. Epitools Epidemiological Calculators. Ausvet. Available online: http://epitools.ausvet.com.au. (accessed on 15 June 2020).
67. McHugh, M.L. Interrater reliability: The kappa statistic. *Biochem. Med.* **2012**, *22*, 276–282. [CrossRef]

pathogens

MDPI

Article

Monitoring *Mycoplasma bovis* Diversity and Antimicrobial Susceptibility in Calf Feedlots Undergoing a Respiratory Disease Outbreak

Claire A.M. Becker [1,*], Chloé Ambroset [1], Anthéa Huleux [2,†], Angélique Vialatte [2,‡], Adélie Colin [2], Agnès Tricot [1], Marie-Anne Arcangioli [1] and Florence Tardy [2]

1 UMR Mycoplasmoses des Ruminants, VetAgro Sup, Université de Lyon, 69280 Marcy-l'Etoile, France; chloe.ambroset@vetagro-sup.fr (C.A.); agnes.tricot@vetagro-sup.fr (A.T.); marie-anne.arcangioli@vetagro-sup.fr (M.-A.A.)

2 UMR Mycoplasmoses des Ruminants, ANSES Laboratoire de Lyon, Université de Lyon, 69364 Lyon CEDEX 07, France; anthea.huleux@orange.fr (A.H.); angelique.vialatte@gmail.com (A.V.); adelie.colin@anses.fr (A.C.); florence.tardy@anses.fr (F.T.)

* Correspondence: claire.becker@vetagro-sup.fr

† Current Address: Cancer Research Centre of Lyon, 69008 Lyon, France.

‡ Current Address: Mylan Laboratories SAS, 01400 Châtillon-sur-Chalaronne, France.

Received: 30 June 2020; Accepted: 11 July 2020; Published: 21 July 2020

Abstract: Bovine respiratory diseases (BRD) are widespread in veal calf feedlots. Several pathogens are implicated, both viruses and bacteria, one of which, *Mycoplasma bovis*, is under-researched. This worldwide-distributed bacterium has been shown to be highly resistant in vitro to the main antimicrobials used to treat BRD. Our objective was to monitor the relative prevalence of *M. bovis* during BRD episodes, its diversity, and its resistance phenotype in relation to antimicrobial use. For this purpose, a two-year longitudinal follow-up of 25 feedlots was organized and 537 nasal swabs were collected on 358 veal calves at their arrival in the lot, at the BRD peak and 4 weeks after collective antimicrobial treatments. The presence of *M. bovis* was assessed by real-time PCR and culture. The clones isolated were then subtyped (*polC* subtyping and PFGE analysis), and their susceptibility to five antimicrobials was determined. The course of the disease and the antimicrobials used had no influence on the genetic diversity of the *M. bovis* strains: The subtype distribution was the same throughout the BRD episode and similar to that already described in France, with a major narrowly-variable subtype circulating, st2. The same conclusion holds for antimicrobial resistance (AMR) phenotypes: All the clones were already multiresistant to the main antimicrobials used (except for fluoroquinolones) prior to any treatments. By contrast, changes of AMR phenotypes could be suspected for Pasteurellaceae in two cases in relation to the treatments registered.

Keywords: *Mycoplasma bovis*; antimicrobial resistance; Bovine Respiratory Disease; genetic diversity

1. Introduction

Bovine Respiratory Disease (BRD), also known as "shipping fever", is a very common and extremely costly disease impacting the beef cattle industry worldwide [1]. It is a complex viral and/or bacterial infection affecting the upper or lower respiratory tracts in cattle, with a particularly high prevalence in recently weaned calves within the first days or weeks of arrival at the feedlot [2]. Multiple stress factors (weaning, transportation, co-mingling in lots or in markets, changes in diet, weather changes, etc.) with additive effects are known to influence the susceptibility of calves to developing BRD [3]. The percentage of morbidity and mortality can reach 70% but varies with the management system in place, prevention programs and the kind of pathogens involved, bacteria being more often fatal than viruses alone [1]. The disease most often results from an overwhelming, dysregulated host immune response [4]. Classical clinical signs of bacterial BRD include fever over 40 °C, dyspnea, nasal discharge, coughing and depression with diminished or no appetite [2]. The most common viral agents associated with BRD include Bovine Herpes Virus type 1 (BHV-1), Parainfluenza-3 virus (PI3), Bovine Viral Diarrhea Virus (BVDV), Bovine Coronavirus (BCoV) and Bovine Respiratory Syncytial Virus (BRSV). The main bacteria are *Mannheimia haemolytica, Pasteurella multocida, Histophilus somni* and *Mycoplasma (M.) bovis* [5,6]. These agents are not all equivalent in terms of pathogenesis, duration of the clinical disease or shedding after exposure [5,6]. Viral agents are thought to be mainly initiators of the disease that then facilitate colonization by bacterial pathogens or aggravating factors during co-infection [7]. Among bacteria, *M. bovis* is still regarded as the least well-characterized BRD pathogen [6–8]. It has been reported to rapidly proliferate in the nasopharynx within the first 14 days of feedlot placement as a preliminary step in the development of BRD [3,9]. Asymptomatic carriage months or even years after an outbreak have been described but with a low prevalence and a role on transmission yet to be defined [10].

Prevention and control of BRD rely on metaphylaxis in high-risk herds (e.g., >1000 animals in the USA), bacterial vaccinations when available, but with controversial efficacies, and antimicrobial treatments of diseased animals [11,12]. Because feedlot management uses many antimicrobials, antimicrobial resistance (AMR) among the bacterial pathogens commonly associated with BRD has been increasingly reported worldwide [12,13]. *M. bovis* is no exception [14].

In France, previous studies have demonstrated the spread of an *M. bovis* clonal population with acquired resistance to most antimicrobial families except for fluoroquinolones [15–17]. However, these data capture a particular context of sampling that might not reflect the short-term evolution of isolates toward AMR. All these studies used strains collected in the framework of our network, Vigimyc, a "passive" surveillance network, the decision to test for mycoplasmas being solely on the initiative of the veterinarian [18]. Most often, a diagnosis for *Mycoplasma* is requested when all other analyses have proved negative or when a treatment failure is observed. Biased sampling might therefore result from using Vigimyc strains as they often originate from antimicrobials-treated animals. *Mycoplasma* species are known to evolve fast, and they develop AMR mainly through mutations in antimicrobial targets, which could be rapidly selected under antimicrobial pressure [19–22].

The present study was conducted to refine our understanding of relationships between antimicrobial use, AMR phenotype (as Minimum inhibitory concentration, MIC) and clonal diversity in *M. bovis* during BRD episodes. For that purpose, a longitudinal follow-up of 25 feedlots was conducted, with complete etiological exploration when BRD cases occurred, from the day of introduction to 4 weeks after the clinical peak. *M. bovis* isolate diversity per feedlot and per animal (by molecular subtyping and Pulsed-Field Gel Electrophoresis, PFGE) and AMR were analyzed before and after treatments. The relative persistence of *M. bovis* and Pasteurellaceae after antimicrobial treatment was also explored.

2. Results

2.1. M. bovis Was the Third Most Frequently Isolated Pathogen (in Association with Others) in Calf Feedlots at BRD Onset

During the 2016–2017 and 2017–2018 winters, 537 double nasal swabs (DNS) were sampled on 358 veal calves in 25 feedlots of Western France. Their characteristics are listed in Supplementary Table S1. Three sampling times were defined: introduction of the animals (T0), BRD peak (T1) and 4 weeks after collective antimicrobial treatment (T2) (Figure 1, Table 1). Four feedlots were excluded from the prevalence study as no BRD episode occurred.

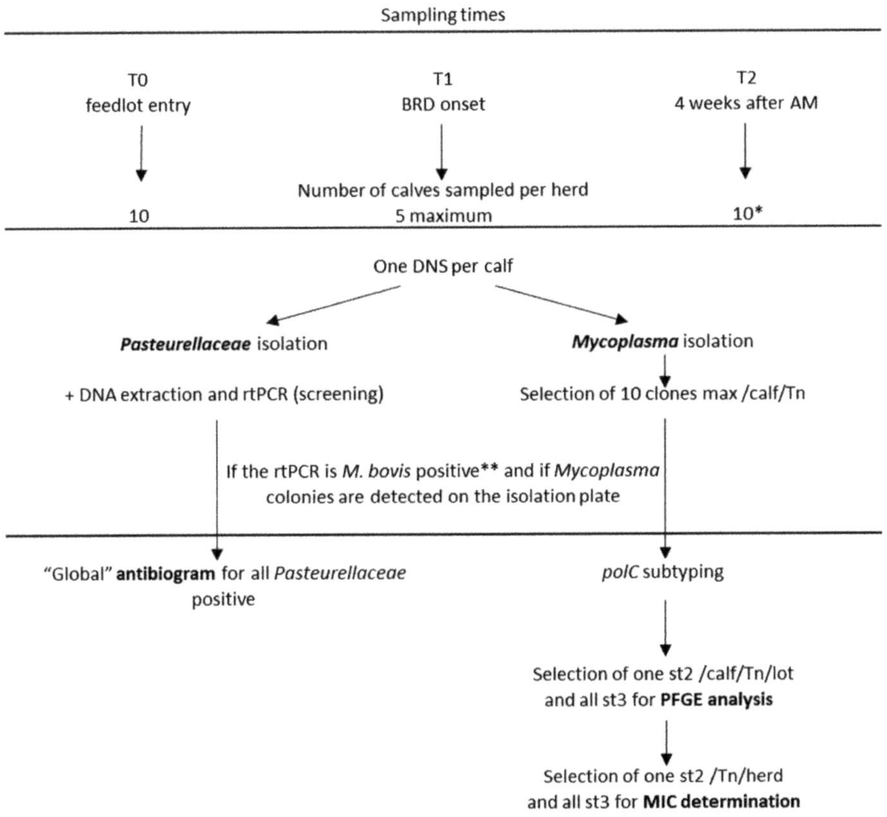

Figure 1. Workflow for sample collection and analyses. DNS, double nasal swab; AM, antimicrobial treatment. * If possible the same 10 calves were sampled at T0 and T2. ** Ct ≤ 37 in rtPCR.

Table 1. Number of double nasal swabs (DNS), calves harboring *M. bovis* (assessed with culture and real-time Polymerase Chain Reaction (rtPCR)) and clones isolated at each sampling time.

	T0	T1	T2	Total
DNS	271	115	151	537
Calves with *M. bovis* rtPCR	6 (2%)	59 (51%)	39/79 * (49%)	104
Calves with *M. bovis* culture	5 (2%)	60 (52%)	28 (19%)	93
Isolated clones	38	251	125	414

T0, feedlot entry; T1, BRD onset; T2, 4 weeks after antimicrobial treatment. * Not all T2 samples were tested by rtPCR (see Supplementary Table S1 for details).

At BRD onset (T1), the etiology was determined using a real-time Polymerase Chain Reaction (rtPCR) screening of seven pathogens (Figure 2). Out of the 21 feedlots where BRD occurred, 115 calves were tested, and *M. bovis* was detected in 51% of them (n = 59), with a mean Ct of 25.7 [20.4–35]. The positive calves (Ct ≤ 37) originated from 18 feedlots: Three feedlots had only calves negative for *M. bovis* (Supplementary Table S1). *M. bovis* ranked as the third most prevalent pathogen after *P. multocida* and the Coronavirus, this triple association being the most common coinfection, calves being frequently infected by more than one pathogen. The proportion of calves found positive at T1 by a culture approach was very similar to that from rtPCR (52%, n = 60) (Table 1). We note that for some calves in different lots (e.g., ME, Supplementary Table S1), cultures were initially positive for *M. bovis*, but no clones could be successfully retrieved from plates, mainly due to coinfections with *M. bovirhinis*.

By contrast, *M. bovis* was seldom detected at feedlot entry (T0). Detection rate was 2%: 5/271 calves by culture and 6/271 by rtPCR, with a mean Ct of 36.7 [25.4–36.8], this difference being compatible with a weak infectious load in the positive calves. Four weeks after the antimicrobial treatment (T2), the presence of *M. bovis* remained high as determined by rtPCR (49%, 39/79, 12/13 feedlots being positive (Supplementary Table S1) with a mean Ct of 30.4 [23.6–36.7]. These Ct values suggest that at this stage of clinical recovery, the viable *Mycoplasma* load was rather low, as the proportion of calves positive by culture was only 17% (25/151 calves, 13/24 lots being considered positive, see Supplementary Table S1).

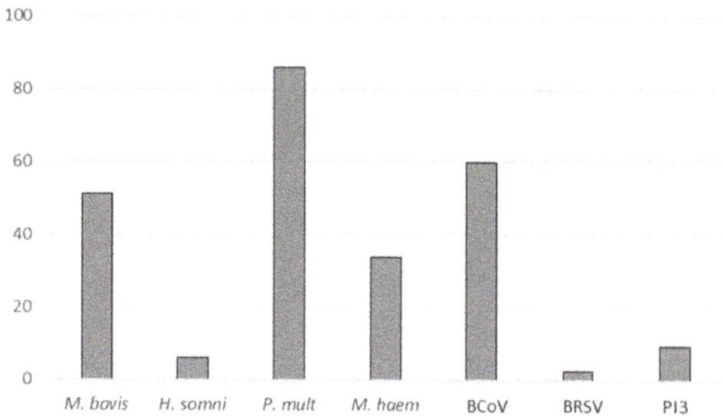

Figure 2. Proportions of calves harboring the different pathogens as assessed by rtPCR at BRD onset (T1, n = 115 calves tested).

The different pathogens tested, indicated on x-axis, are *Mycoplasma bovis* (*M. bovis*), *Histophilus somni* (*H. somni*), *Pasteurella multocida* (*P. mult*), *Mannheimia haemolytica* (*M. haem*), Bovine Coronavirus (BCoV), Bovine Respiratory Syncytial Virus (BRSV) and Parainfluenza 3 virus (PI3). Y-axis, percentage of calves infected with each pathogen.

2.2. The Diversity of Clones Does Not Differ at Different Sampling Times and Is Similar to the Reference Population of Vigimyc Isolates

The number of isolated clones per feedlot (with a maximum of 10 per calf) selected from agar plates, with their characteristics, is given in Supplementary Table S1. Out of the 414 clones retrieved from the 93 calves sampled at different times in the 25 feedlots, 400 were subtyped using the *polC* subtyping scheme as proposed earlier [15]. Most (313/400, 78%) st2 was recovered, but st3 was also present (86/400, 21%). Both subtypes could be found in the same feedlot at the same sampling time, but no calf was shown to harbor both subtypes at one sampling time. For this reason, we further analyzed the proportion of subtypes per calf at each sampling time, which we considered thereafter as our epidemiological unit. This proportion was of 81% calves having a st2 *M. bovis* (Figure 3A), while 18% had a st3 *M. bovis*. Surprisingly, a new st was defined in the French scheme for one calf (T2-RO-1647, black on Figure 3) showing 15 SNPs with respect to the reference sequence of $PG45^{TS}$ (11 out of 15 SNPs in common with the st3 sequence). The subtype determined using the MLST scheme of Register was ST45 (legacy scheme, ST124) [23,24].

The st proportions were identical between different sampling times (Figure 3B). No clear evolution of subtypes proportions was observed along the study, whatever the antimicrobials used in the herds (Supplementary Table S2). Some calves harbored the same st in T1 and T2 (e.g., HA-8680 with st2 or NE-6423 with st3), whereas others had a different st at the two sampling times (e.g., NE-8907 st2 then st3 or CA-8149 st3 then st2), suggesting a potential contamination by another strain in the course of the fattening period.

The overall proportions of the st in the study (calculated on calf numbers) was compared to the diversity retrieved among the strains of the Vigimyc network over the past six years (Figure 3A). The same epidemiological tendency was observed between the study strains and the Vigimyc strains: The st2 *polC* subtype was the most prevalent, while the proportion of st3 was similar at each sampling date in this study (19%).

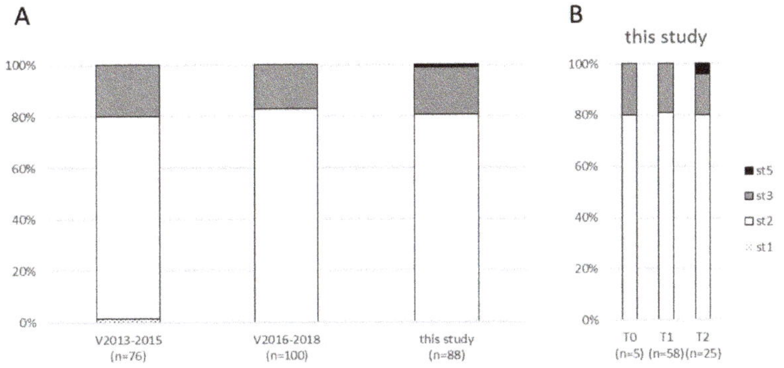

Figure 3. Subtype proportions of French strains of the Vigimyc network over the past 6 years and the clones of this study determined by *polC* subtyping. (**A**) Global comparison between Vigimyc strains and those from the present study and (**B**) detailed proportions of st according to sampling times (T0, T1, T2) in this study. X-axis, category of strains (Vigimyc, V, with different sampling year or this study); y-axis, proportion of each subtype. Numbers in brackets under each lane indicate the number of strains tested.

A restricted panel of clones was then analyzed by PFGE to further evaluate their relatedness. We first evaluated intra-st2 diversity by analyzing all the clones from two feedlots. All the st2 clones retrieved from eight sampled calves showed a unique, identical PFGE pattern, with no difference between calves or feedlots (data not shown). Consequently, in further analyses, for st2, only one clone per calf and per sampling time was selected. Because an increased diversity was expected from st3 clones [15] and as these were less numerous, they were all tested by PFGE. The PFGE patterns were homogeneous for all the st2 clones (Branch A in Figure 4) while the st3 clones showed more diversity (Branches B to I, in Figure 4, see also Supplementary Table S2). This within-st3 diversity was observed at different levels, i.e., different feedlots, different calves, or even different clones isolated from the same calf (e.g., T1-FO-0494-c3 or c11 * in Figure 4). However, no correlation was established between the PFGE profiles and the treatment history or sampling date. The st5 clone was found in a specific, different branch (J in Figure 4), showing a more distant profile.

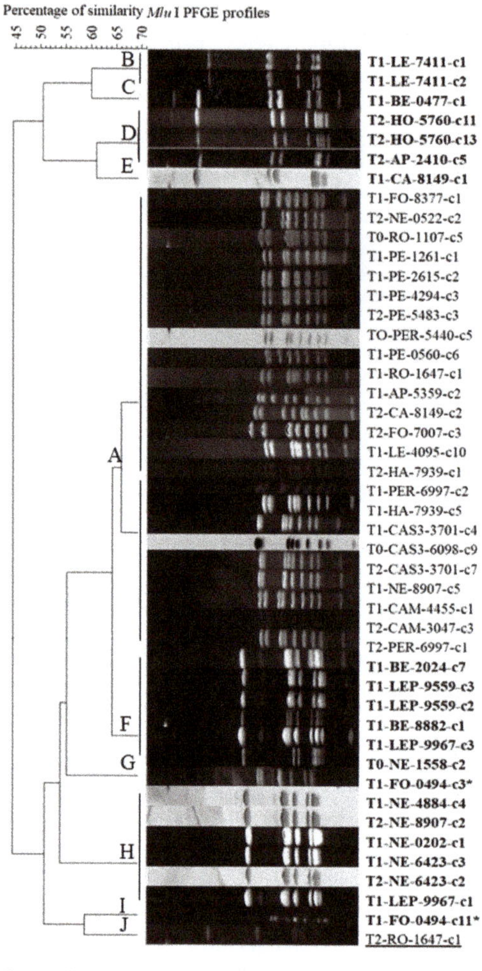

Figure 4. Cluster analysis of 46 *M. bovis* clones based on their Pulse Field Gel Electrophoresis (PFGE)-*MluI* profiles using the Dice coefficient and UPGMA method. The resulting degree of similarity is indicated on the scale on the top left corner (similarity cut-off value set at 70%). *M. bovis* clones are characterized by the sampling time, feedlot name, calf number and clone number. (**A**) cluster of st2 strains; (**B–I**) clusters of st3 strains (bold); J, branch for the clone of new st5 (underlined); the asterisk indicates 2 clones coming from the same calf with different PFGE profiles.

2.3. *M. bovis Field Isolates Are Already Multiresistant to Antimicrobials before Any Treatment in the Lot*

Antimicrobial susceptibility was tested on 39 clones representative of the various genetic subtypes or macrorestriction profiles and the different sampling times, i.e., one representative clone of st2 per feedlot and per sampling time and one representative clone per PFGE cluster per calf and per sampling time for st3 (see Supplementary Table S2). As no breakpoints are available for *M. bovis*, clinical breakpoints for Pasteurellaceae were used for interpretation of the results [25] and the MIC90 for the French *M. bovis* population (as calculated from Gautier Bouchardon et al., 2014 for recent isolates, collected between 2010 and 2012 [16]) are also indicated (blue double arrows in Figure 5). Whatever the sampling time, all the clones were resistant to oxytetracycline, tilmicosin and florfenicol (Figure 5A,B,D), except for one susceptible and three intermediary strains for florfenicol (Figure 5D).

By contrast, most of the clones showed a low MIC of enrofloxacin (≤0.25 µg/mL, Figure 5C), except for three clones with a slight increase in MIC (0.5–1 µg/mL). These three clones were isolated from three different feedlots (see Supplementary Table S1): in one of these, oxolinic acid was used once to treat some calves before T1. No relationship was observed between MIC and sampling time, or with subtype.

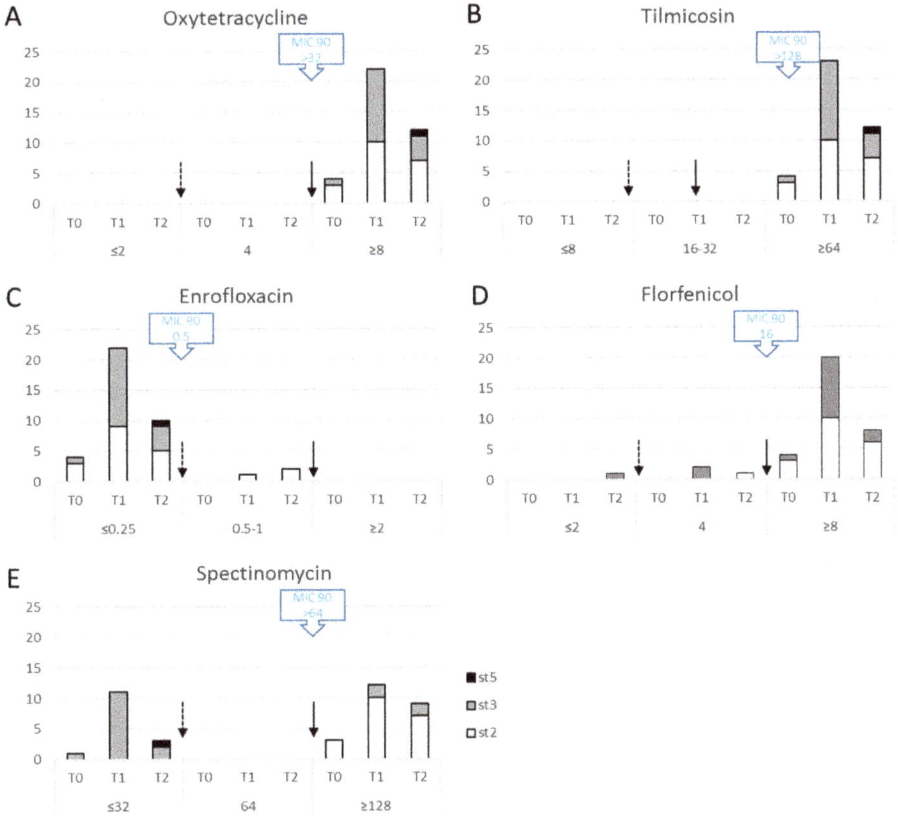

Figure 5. Minimum Inhibitory Concentrations (MICs) for 5 antimicrobial molecules for 39 clones according to their genetic st (*polC* subtyping) and sampling date. (**A**) Oxytetracycline, (**B**) Tilmicosin, (**C**) Enrofloxacin, (**D**) Florfenicol, (**E**) Spectinomycin. X-axis, MIC classes detailed with sampling times; y-axis, number of isolates. Arrows indicate the threshold for Pasteurellaceae when available; dotted arrow, susceptible to intermediate MIC; plain arrow, intermediate to resistant MIC. Blue rectangles with arrow indicate the MIC90 for the French *M. bovis* strains collected between 2010–2012 [16] (oxytetracycline > 32, tilmicosin > 128, enrofloxacin 0.5, florfenicol 16, spectinomycin > 64).

For spectinomycin, 15/39 strains showed surprisingly low MICs (Figure 5E) that classify them as susceptible according to CLSI [25]. They were from T0, T1 or T2 but showed the common characteristic of being of st3 (in one case st5). This contrasted with previous data obtained on French strains (MIC90 > 64 µg/mL for strains collected in 2010–2012 [16]). To further analyze this discrepancy, 33 strains isolated between 2011 and 2018 (mainly st3 and a few st2 as control, see Supplementary Table S1) through the Vigimyc network were selected and their MICs for spectinomycin analyzed (Figure 6). A third of the strains (33.3%) were susceptible to spectinomycin, irrespective of subtype.

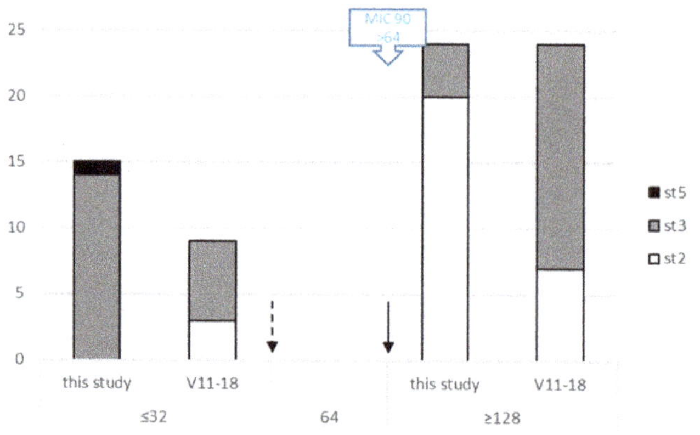

Figure 6. Distribution of *M. bovis* strains MICs for spectinomycin as a function of their origin and genetic subtype (*polC* subtyping). X-axis, spectinomycin MICs for sets of strains (either from Vigimyc and isolated between 2011 to 2018, V11-18, or from this study); y-axis, number of isolates. Arrows indicate the threshold for Pasteurellaceae when available; dotted arrow, susceptible to intermediate MIC; plain arrow, intermediate to resistant MIC. Blue rectangle with arrow indicates the MIC90 for the French *M. bovis* strains collected between 2010–2012 [16] (spectinomycin > 64).

No correlation could be found between antimicrobial treatments used in the feedlots (Supplementary Table S1) and either MIC or genetic subtype, whatever the substance used. No selection was observed as a result of the various treatments used in the feedlots.

2.4. Antimicrobial Resistance Profile of Pasteurellaceae Is Different from That of M. bovis

M. bovis and Pasteurellaceae were co-isolated in 13 occurrences (five different feedlots, different sampling times) (see Supplementary Table S2 and Figure S1). In these 13 occurrences of co-isolation, the antimicrobial susceptibility profiles of Pasteurellaceae were examined by the disk method. *P. multocida* strains were mainly sensitive to amoxicillin, tulathromycin, tylosin, spectinomycin, florfenicol, enrofloxacin and marbofloxacin but resistant to tetracycline. In one feedlot (CAM) we detected strains resistant to tulathromycin. The sole strain of *M. haemolytica* that was isolated in the study (T1, herd NE) was resistant to amoxicillin, intermediate for enrofloxacin and tulathromycin and susceptible for the other antimicrobials.

In two feedlots (CAS5 and NE), collective antimicrobial treatments could have helped to select resistant strains. In CAS5 where doxycycline was used as metaphylaxis at the BRD peak, isolates were resistant to tetracycline at T1 and T2 but not at T0 (Supplementary Figure S1A,D). In NE, where spectinomycin was used individually, though not for the sampled calves, isolates were resistant to spectinomycin at T1 and T2 but not at T0 (Supplementary Figure S1E).

Pasteurellaceae remained globally largely more susceptible to antimicrobials than *M. bovis*. Although it is hard to conclude on a small number of strains, it seems that treatment influenced Pasteurellaceae antimicrobial susceptibility patterns, as the selection of resistant isolates was observed in two situations.

3. Discussion

In the present study, out of 25 monitored feedlots, 21 experienced a BRD episode, of which 18 were positive for *M. bovis*, among other pathogens, at the disease peak (T1). This high prevalence confirms the major contribution of *M. bovis* in BRD in this context of feedlots where animals of several origins are comingled [26]. *M. bovis* was most often associated with other pathogens, such as *P. multocida* and the Coronavirus (Figure 2), also frequently reported in BRD episodes [3,27]. Nevertheless, these prevalence results may be related to our sampling choice, i.e., nasal swabs. The Bovine Coronavirus was indeed shown to be detected in higher proportions in superficial samplings than in the lower respiratory tract samples, such as bronchoalveolar lavages [28]. The overall mycoplasmal load per calf was high at the disease peak, with a mean Ct of 25.7. Nonetheless, in 2/4 feedlots with no BRD episode, we were able to detect *M. bovis*-positive calves at T2, suggesting a potential asymptomatic circulation of the pathogen in the absence of any clinical disease as already suggested [8]. The weak prevalence observed at T0 (2% of positive calves) seems a true picture of the actual circulation of *M. bovis* in dairy herds in France [29], calves reared in feedlots mainly coming from dairy herds.

Four weeks after antimicrobial treatment (T2), when acute clinical signs of BRD were over, 49% of the calves remained rtPCR-positive for *M. bovis* against 51% at T1, indicating failed microbial clearance by treatments. However, the increase in the mean Ct to 30.4 and the low proportion of calves tested positive by culture (19%) suggest that at this stage of clinical recovery, the viable *Mycoplasma* load was significantly reduced. At T2, the proportion of *M. bovis*-positive animals estimated by culture was comparable to that recorded by our epidemiosurveillance network Vigimyc (15%, [18]). This suggests that most often, in day to day diagnosis, mycoplasmas are searched for only after antimicrobial treatment, remaining an etiology explored in case of failure of clinical improvement after chemotherapy.

We further showed that the overall genetic diversity of strains, assessed by *polC* subtyping [15] and PFGE analysis [30], was unmodified either by the ongoing BRD episode or by the associated antimicrobial treatments. The proportion of the two main *polC* subtypes currently circulating in France was comparable at each sampling time (feedlot entry, BRD peak and 4 weeks after the peak), i.e., 80% st2 and 20% st3. This proportion was also comparable to that of diagnosis strains collected in the framework of the Vigimyc surveillance network [15]. This confirms that our network, in its current operating procedures [18], is able to collect strains representative of those circulating in France and so is a real resource for monitoring genetic diversity and AMR.

PFGE patterns confirmed that st3 strains were more variable than st2 strains [15], but once again, this diversity was not related to any particular evolution of BRD or antimicrobial treatments. Both subtypes could be found circulating in the same herd, although no calf was detected harboring both subtypes at any one time. Considering the marked polymorphisms between st2 and st3, it is unlikely that the switch of subtypes observed on some calves over time (from T1 to T2, st2→st3 or st3→st2) could result from genetic evolution of the strains in such a short interval. The most likely scenario is co-circulation within a lot or a calf of the two subtypes, a possibility not observed here but previously reported and one becoming more prevalent at the time of sampling. Interestingly, a different subtype, never detected before in France, namely st5, was found in the RO feedlot. It had already been described in North America (ST124, in the legacy MLST scheme or ST45 in the revised scheme of Register [31,32]). Further genomic and phylogenetic characterization of this strain is ongoing, especially to establish phylogenetic relationships between the three subtypes.

As expected from studies around the world, our MIC data confirmed the overall multiresistance of *M. bovis* strains. For all the antimicrobials, resistance levels were the same as reported recently elsewhere [12,33–41]: *M. bovis* strains were resistant to tetracyclines, macrolides and florfenicol (with a few intermediate strains). However, we were further able to demonstrate that strains were already resistant before any antimicrobial treatment and that their MIC patterns were not changed in the course of the BRD episode and the associated chemotherapy. These results show that resistant clones are not selected during the disease episode but that clones circulating in France are already multiresistant. Fluoroquinolones remain the only antimicrobials with low MICs, which might be due to their restricted use in veterinary medicine owing to their classification as critically important antimicrobials. For this family, although we could fear an MIC increase for st3 due to a greater ability to fix mutations in vitro under subinhibitory concentrations of enrofloxacin [19], we observed the same susceptibility profiles for both subtypes. The few strains showing a slight increase in MIC of enrofloxacin to an intermediate level were st2, most strains of both subtypes being susceptible. The hypothesis of the spread since the year 2000 of a dominant multiresistant clone is thus confirmed [15] and we further rule out the possibility of the co-existence of susceptible clones.

The situation was different for Pasteurellaceae, for which we were partly able to correlate antimicrobial treatments and change in susceptibility profiles. We managed to gather data on antimicrobial use, although stockbreeders did not always continuously record treatments, which resulted in some incomplete data [40] (Supplementary Table S2). However, potential acquisition of AMR was recorded in two feedlots (CAS5 and NE), where the targeted antimicrobials had been used. This underlines the fact that acquisition of AMR may not have the same dynamics for *M. bovis* and for Pasteurellaceae. For the latter, AMR may arise during the BRD course under the influence of chemotherapy as already demonstrated by the apparition or spreading of new clones [42]. We were able to illustrate this fact only in two herds, because of the difficulty to retrieve Pasteurellaceae from nasal swabs that are often polymicrobial [43].

One unexpected finding in this study was the diversity of susceptibility profiles for spectinomycin, contrasting with previous observations that classified *M. bovis* as 100% resistant to this drug in France [16]. The decrease in spectinomycin MICs in France could signal a reappearance of more susceptible profiles, which are observed elsewhere in the world [33,34]. This mixed situation, with the coexistence of highly and poorly spectinomycin-resistant strains is very similar to what has been described in Hungary [38]. It would be of interest to investigate whether it is associated with a true reversion of antimicrobial resistance genotypes, with notably mutations (and reversions) in the *rrs* genes at position 1192 as previously reported [22,34].

4. Materials and Methods

4.1. Sampling Campaigns

A total of 537 veal calves were sampled in 25 fattening units located in Western France from November to April 2016–2017 and November to April 2017–2018. The size of each feedlot, ranging from 22 to 519 heads, and the antimicrobial treatments used during the observation periods were recorded (for more details see Supplementary Tables S1 and S2). Figure 1 summarizes the sampling and analysis workflow. In each herd, 10 randomly chosen calves were sampled using double nasal swabs (DNS) when introduced in the feedlot (T0). When a BRD episode occurred in the feedlot and before any collective antimicrobial treatment (T1), DNS were taken from five diseased calves. Four weeks after the end of the collective antimicrobial treatment (T2), the ten calves sampled at T0 were re-sampled, if possible. All DNS (T0, T1, T2) were sent, dry, at 4 °C, within at most two days after sampling, to the Anses laboratory. One swab was used for Pasteurellaceae isolation on Columbia agar plate containing 5% sheep blood (Biomérieux) and then for nucleic acid extraction (see hereafter). Another swab was used for *Mycoplasma* isolation (see below).

4.2. Nucleic Acid Extraction from Swabs and rtPCR Amplifications

Nucleic acids were extracted from swabs using the simplified protocol described previously [44]. Briefly, swabs were squeezed and sterilely cut in a tube containing a lysis buffer (TRIS 0.1 M, Tween 20 0.05% and proteinase K 0.24 mg/mL). They were heated for 1 h at 60 °C and then for 15 min at 95 °C to inactivate the proteinase. Real-time PCR (rtPCR) was performed on these bulk extracts using LSI VetMAX Screening pack Ruminant Respiratory Pathogens (ThermoFisher) to detect the various pathogens responsible for BRD (*M. bovis*, *Histophilus somni*, *Pasteurella multocida*, *Mannheimia haemolytica*, Coronavirus, Respiratory Syncytial Virus and Parainfluenza 3) (at T1), or with VetMAX™ *M. bovis* Kit (ThermoFisher) to only assess *M. bovis* presence (at T0 and T2), according to the manufacturer's recommendations. The Ct cut-off for *M. bovis*-positiveness was set at ≤ 37 according to the recommendation of Wisselink et al. [45].

4.3. Isolation and Identification of *M. bovis* Isolates

Swabs were seeded on plates containing a PPLO agar medium modified as previously described [46], with addition of 0.1% of Tween 80 for specific inhibition of *M. bovirhinis* potential contamination [47]. Plates were incubated for 4 days at 37 °C in 5% CO_2. A maximum of 10 clones per calf and per sampling point were randomly selected with a wooden toothpick, further cultured in 2 mL PPLO broth and identified using membrane filtration dot-immunobinding tests (MF-Dot) as previously described [48]. As the number of picked clones per calf varied with the quality of the isolation, each calf at one sampling time (T0, T1 or T2) was considered as a single epidemiological unit.

A set of *M. bovis* isolates from a collection kept at Anses, Lyon Laboratory and mostly derived from the French national surveillance network for mycoplasmosis in ruminants (Vigimyc) [18] were included in the study as a "reference" population for both subtyping and antimicrobial resistance.

4.4. Strain Subtyping by Sequence Analysis of the Housekeeping Gene polC and Pulse Field Gel Electrophoresis (PFGE)

Genomic DNA was extracted from 200 μL of each clone culture using QIAamp® DNA Minikit (Qiagen), and the *M. bovis* clones were all subtyped using *polC* sequence analysis as previously described [15] (Figure 1).

One isolate yielded a new *polC* subtype and was further analyzed to determine its subtype according to the MLST scheme of Register et al. ([24]; https://pulmlst.org/bovis/), by a whole genome resequencing approach. Briefly, a DNA sample was sequenced using an Illumina MiSeq technology generating 2 × 300-bp pair-end reads (MiSeq 600 cycles V3 kit, Biofidal, Vaux-en-Velin, France). A total of 1,443,759 reads were generated for each R*, resulting in an average coverage of 860 X. Trimmed reads (using Trimmomatic-0.36) were aligned to two reference genomes, namely PG45 (refseq NC_014760.1) and JF4278 (a corrected version provided by Bern University).

After quality control of the alignments, the variants were identified and annotated using GATK4 v4.0.10.0 (https://software.broadinstitute.org/gatk). The filtered output vcf files were then used to retrieve the different Register loci sequences [24].

A sub-panel of clones was selected (one st2 per calf at each sampling time and per lot and all st3, Figure 1 and Supplementary Table S1) to be further subtyped by Pulse-Field Gel Electrophoresis (PFGE) with the *MluI* enzyme as previously described [30]. Briefly, mycoplasma cells from overnight cultures were embedded in low melt agarose plugs and lysed by proteinase K before DNA overnight restriction using endonucleases. The macrorestriction fragments were separated by electrophoresis on a CHEF-DR III system (Bio-Rad) in 1% agarose gel, in TBE 0.5% at 14 °C, for 24h, with an included angle of 120°. Images were analyzed with the software Bionumerics GelCompar II v6.6 (Applied Maths NV, Sint-Martens-Latem, Belgium). The similarity analysis was carried out using the Dice coefficient (position tolerance 1.5%) and a dendrogram was constructed using the UPGMA method.

4.5. Antimicrobial Susceptibility Testing of *M. bovis* and Pasteurellaceae

The susceptibility of the selected *M. bovis* clones was tested using Minimum inhibitory concentration (MICs) assays as previously described [17] for the five antimicrobial classes mostly used to treat BRD in the field and known to be potentially active against *Mycoplasma* spp: quinolones (enrofloxacin), tetracyclines (oxytetracycline), phenicols (florfenicol), aminoglycosides (spectinomycin) and macrolides (tilmicosin). Briefly, clones were plated on PPLO agar plates containing twofold increasing antimicrobial concentrations, either as a full range of antimicrobial dilutions or only for a few concentrations corresponding to the CLSI clinical breakpoints for Pasteurellaceae, a family known to colonize the same body niche [25]. At least two experiments were conducted, and the modes of the different results were retained as the final MIC values. For some strains, the different experiments did not allow us to conclude on a single MIC value: an MIC interval was defined (Supplementary Table S2) but was not represented in Figure 5.

Antibiograms for Pasteurellaceae were outsourced at the Laboratoire Vétérinaire Départemental du Rhône. For each sample positive for both *M. bovis* and Pasteurellaceae, a mix of Pasteurellaceae-like colonies with similar phenotype was collected from the Columbia agar plate, identified with an API 20E gallery and tested for resistance with the standardized diffusion method in agar (norm NF U47-107) for the same five antimicrobial classes tested for *M. bovis* (depending on the available disks): quinolones (enrofloxacin and marbofloxacin), tetracyclines (tetracycline), phenicols (florfenicol), aminoglycosides (spectinomycin) and macrolides (tylosin and tulathromycin). The β-lactam amoxicillin known to be active against Pasteurellaceae was also tested. Zone diameters were interpreted according to the CLSI standards [25].

5. Conclusions

This study demonstrates that *M. bovis* is an important player in feedlot BRD. Its prevalence is weak at entry but rapidly increases to reach a peak at the disease onset. It can circulate in the absence of clinical episodes and remain present even after antimicrobial treatments, which can result in clinical recovery without mycoplasmal clearance. The disease course and the associated chemotherapy did not affect the genetic diversity or AMR patterns of strains circulating in a lot. The strains observed in this longitudinal study reflected the general population circulating in France, with one major clone multiresistant to the main antimicrobials used in BRD, also retrieved by our surveillance network.

Supplementary Materials: The following are available online at http://www.mdpi.com/2076-0817/9/7/593/s1, Figure S1: Comparative evolution of zone diameters for the Pasteurellaceae strains before (T1) and 4 weeks after antimicrobial treatment (T2). Table S1: Characteristics of the feedlots. Table S2: Characteristics of the clones studied.

Author Contributions: F.T., M.-A.A., C.B. designed the study. M.-A.A. and F.T. supervised the sampling campaign. A.C., A.H., A.T., A.V., C.A. and C.A.M.B. did the experiments. C.A., C.A.M.B. and F.T. analyzed the results and drafted the manuscript. C.A.M.B. and F.T. reviewed and edited the manuscript. All the authors reviewed the manuscript. All authors have read and agreed to the published version of the manuscript.

Funding: This study was funded by the French Ministry for Agriculture and Food, as an EcoAntibio project.

Acknowledgments: The authors are grateful to the veterinarians who sampled the calves and gave access to antimicrobial treatment data. Special thanks go to François Poumarat and Maryne Jaÿ, respectively former and current manager of Vigimyc, who made surveillance data available.

Conflicts of Interest: All the authors declare they have no competing interests for this study.

References

1. Urban-Chmiel, R.; Grooms, D.L. Prevention and Control of Bovine Respiratory Disease. *J. Livest. Sci.* **2012**, *3*, 27–36.
2. Snowder, G.D.; Van Vleck, L.D.; Cundiff, L.V.; Bennett, G.L. Bovine respiratory disease in feedlot cattle: Environmental, genetic, and economic factors. *J. Anim. Sci.* **2006**, *84*, 1999–2008. [CrossRef]
3. Cirone, F.; Padalino, B.; Tullio, D.; Capozza, P.; Losurdo, M.; Lanave, G.; Pratelli, A. Prevalence of Pathogens Related to Bovine Respiratory Disease Before and After Transportation in Beef Steers: Preliminary Results. *Animals* **2019**, *9*, 1093. [CrossRef] [PubMed]
4. McGill, J.L.; Sacco, R.E. The Immunology of Bovine Respiratory Disease: Recent Advancements. *Vet. Clin. N. Am. Food Anim. Pract.* **2020**, in press. [CrossRef]
5. Grissett, G.P.; White, B.J.; Larson, R.L. Structured Literature Review of Responses of Cattle to Viral and Bacterial Pathogens Causing Bovine Respiratory Disease Complex. *J. Vet. Intern. Med.* **2015**, *29*, 770–780. [CrossRef] [PubMed]
6. Amat, S.; Holman, D.B.; Timsit, E.; Schwinghamer, T.; Alexander, T.W. Evaluation of the Nasopharyngeal Microbiota in Beef Cattle Transported to a Feedlot, With a Focus on Lactic Acid-Producing Bacteria. *Front. Microbiol.* **2019**, *10*, 1988. [CrossRef] [PubMed]
7. Taylor, J.D.; Fulton, R.W.; Lehenbauer, T.W.; Step, D.L.; Confer, A.W. The epidemiology of bovine respiratory disease: What is the evidence for predisposing factors? *Can. Vet. J.* **2010**, *51*, 1095–1102. [PubMed]

8. Maunsell, F.P.; Woolums, A.R.; Francoz, D.; Rosenbusch, R.F.; Step, D.L.; Wilson, D.J.; Janzen, E.D. *Mycoplasma bovis* infections in cattle. *J. Vet. Intern. Med.* **2011**, *25*, 772–783. [CrossRef]
9. Holman, D.B.; Timsit, E.; Amat, S.; Abbott, D.W.; Buret, A.G.; Alexander, T.W. The nasopharyngeal microbiota of beef cattle before and after transport to a feedlot. *BMC Microbiol.* **2017**, *17*, 70. [CrossRef]
10. Calcutt, M.J.; Lysnyansky, I.; Sachse, K.; Fox, L.K.; Nicholas, R.A.J.; Ayling, R.D. Gap analysis of *Mycoplasma bovis* disease, diagnosis and control: An aid to identify future development requirements. *Transbound. Emerg. Dis.* **2018**, *65*, 91–109. [CrossRef]
11. Amat, S.; Timsit, E.; Baines, D.; Yanke, J.; Alexander, T.W. Development of Bacterial Therapeutics against the Bovine Respiratory Pathogen *Mannheimia haemolytica*. *Appl. Environ. Microbiol.* **2019**, *85*, e01359-19. [CrossRef] [PubMed]
12. Stanford, K.; Zaheer, R.; Klima, C.; McAllister, T.; Peters, D.; Niu, Y.D.; Ralston, B. Antimicrobial Resistance in Members of the Bacterial Bovine Respiratory Disease Complex Isolated from Lung Tissue of Cattle Mortalities Managed with or without the Use of Antimicrobials. *Microorganisms* **2020**, *8*, 288. [CrossRef] [PubMed]
13. De Donder, K.D.; Apley, M.D. A Review of the Expected Effects of Antimicrobials in Bovine Respiratory Disease Treatment and Control Using Outcomes from Published Randomized Clinical Trials with Negative Controls. *Vet. Clin. N. Am. Food Anim. Pract.* **2015**, *31*, 97–111. [CrossRef]
14. Gautier-Bouchardon, A.V. Antimicrobial Resistance in *Mycoplasma* spp. *Microbiol. Spectr.* **2018**, 6. [CrossRef]
15. Becker, C.A.M.; Thibault, F.M.; Arcangioli, M.-A.; Tardy, F. Genotypic evolution of *Mycoplasma bovis* isolates collected in France over the last 35 years. In Proceedings of the Progress in Human and Animal Mycoplasmology, Istanbul, Turkey, 3–5 June 2015; p. 60.
16. Gautier-Bouchardon, A.V.; Ferre, S.; Le Grand, D.; Paoli, A.; Gay, E.; Poumarat, F. Overall Decrease in the Susceptibility of *Mycoplasma bovis* to Antimicrobials over the Past 30 Years in France. *PLoS ONE* **2014**, *9*, e87672. [CrossRef]
17. Khalil, D.; Becker, C.A.M.; Tardy, F. Monitoring the decrease in susceptibility to ribosomal RNAs targeting antimicrobials and its molecular basis in clinical *Mycoplasma bovis* isolates over time. *Microb. Drug Resist.* **2017**, *23*, 799–811. [CrossRef]
18. Poumarat, F.; Jarrige, N.; Tardy, F. Principe et bilan du réseau Vigimyc consacré à l'épidémiosurveillance des mycoplasmoses des ruminants en France. *Euroref. Cah. Réf.* **2014**, *12*, 24–29.
19. Khalil, D.; Becker, C.A.M.; Tardy, F. Alterations in the Quinolone Resistance-Determining Regions and Fluoroquinolone Resistance in Clinical Isolates and Laboratory-Derived Mutants of *Mycoplasma bovis*: Not All Genotypes May Be Equal. *Appl. Environ. Microbiol.* **2016**, *82*, 1060–1068. [CrossRef]
20. Sato, T.; Higuchi, H.; Yokota, S.-i.; Tamura, Y. *Mycoplasma bovis* isolates from dairy calves in Japan have less susceptibility than a reference strain to all approved macrolides associated with a point mutation (G748A) combined with multiple species-specific nucleotide alterations in 23S rRNA. *Microbiol. Immunol.* **2017**, *61*, 215–224. [CrossRef]
21. Sato, T.; Okubo, T.; Usui, M.; Higuchi, H.; Tamura, Y. Amino Acid Substitutions in GyrA and ParC Are Associated with Fluoroquinolone Resistance in *Mycoplasma bovis* Isolates from Japanese Dairy Calves. *J. Vet. Med. Sci.* **2013**, *75*, 1063–1065. [CrossRef]
22. Sulyok, K.M.; Kreizinger, Z.; Wehmann, E.; Lysnyansky, I.; Bányai, K.; Marton, S.; Jerzsele, Á.; Rónai, Z.; Turcsányi, I.; Makrai, L.; et al. Mutations Associated with Decreased Susceptibility to Seven Antimicrobial Families in Field and Laboratory-Derived *Mycoplasma bovis* Strains. *Antimicrob. Agents Chemother.* **2017**, 61. [CrossRef] [PubMed]
23. Register, K.B.; Lysnyansky, I.; Jelinski, M.D.; Boatwright, W.D.; Waldner, M.; Bayles, D.O.; Pilo, P.; Alt, D.P. Comparison of Two Multilocus Sequence Typing Schemes for *Mycoplasma bovis* and Revision of the PubMLST Reference Method. *J. Clin. Microbiol.* **2020**, in press. [CrossRef]
24. Register, K.B.; Thole, L.; Rosenbush, R.F.; Minion, F.C. Multilocus sequence typing of *Mycoplasma bovis* reveals host-specific genotypes in cattle versus bison. *Vet. Microbiol.* **2015**, *175*, 92–98. [CrossRef] [PubMed]
25. Clinical and laboratory standards institute. *Performance Standards for Antimicrobial Disk and Dilution Susceptibility Tests for Bacteria Isolated From Animals*, 3rd ed.; Clinical and Laboratory Standards Institute: Wayne, PA, USA, 2015.
26. Caswell, J.L.; Bateman, K.G.; Cai, H.Y.; Castillo-Alcala, F. *Mycoplasma bovis* in respiratory disease of feedlot cattle. *Vet. Clin. N. Am. Food Anim. Pract.* **2010**, *26*, 365–379. [CrossRef] [PubMed]

27. Decaro, N.; Campolo, M.; Desario, C.; Cirone, F.; D'abramo, M.; Lorusso, E.; Greco, G.; Mari, V.; Colaianni, M.L.; Elia, G.; et al. Respiratory Disease Associated with Bovine Coronavirus Infection in Cattle Herds in Southern Italy. *J. Vet. Diagn. Investig.* **2008**, *20*, 28–32. [CrossRef] [PubMed]
28. Doyle, D.; Credille, B.; Lehenbauer, T.W.; Berghaus, R.; Aly, S.S.; Champagne, J.; Blanchard, P.; Crossley, B.; Berghaus, L.; Cochran, S.; et al. Agreement Among 4 Sampling Methods to Identify Respiratory Pathogens in Dairy Calves with Acute Bovine Respiratory Disease. *J. Vet. Intern. Med.* **2017**, *31*, 954–959. [CrossRef]
29. Arcangioli, M.; Chazel, M.; Sellal, E.; Botrel, M.; Bezille, P.; Poumarat, F.; Calavas, D.; Le Grand, D. Prevalence of *Mycoplasma bovis* udder infection in dairy cattle: Preliminary field investigation in southeast France. *N. Z. Vet. J.* **2011**, *59*, 75–78. [CrossRef]
30. Arcangioli, M.A.; Aslan, H.; Tardy, F.; Poumarat, F.; Le Grand, D. The use of pulsed-field gel electrophoresis to investigate the epidemiology of *Mycoplasma bovis* in French calf feedlots. *Vet. J.* **2012**, *192*, 96–100. [CrossRef]
31. Register, K.B.; Jelinski, M.D.; Waldner, M.; Boatwright, W.D.; Anderson, T.K.; Hunter, D.L.; Hamilton, R.G.; Burrage, P.; Shury, T.; Bildfell, R.; et al. Comparison of multilocus sequence types found among North American isolates of *Mycoplasma bovis* from cattle, bison, and deer, 2007–2017. *J. Vet. Diagn. Investig.* **2019**, *31*, 899–904. [CrossRef]
32. Yair, Y.; Borovok, I.; Mikula, I.; Falk, R.; Fox, L.K.; Gophna, U.; Lysnyansky, I. Genomics-based epidemiology of bovine *Mycoplasma bovis* strains in Israel. *BMC Genom.* **2020**, *21*, 70. [CrossRef]
33. Cai, H.Y.; McDowall, R.; Parker, L.; Kaufman, E.I.; Caswell, J.L. Changes in antimicrobial susceptibility profiles of *Mycoplasma bovis* over time. *Can. J. Vet. Res.* **2019**, *83*, 34–41. [PubMed]
34. Hata, E.; Harada, T.; Itoh, M. Relationship between Antimicrobial Susceptibility and Multilocus Sequence Type of *Mycoplasma bovis* Isolates and Development of a Method for Rapid Detection of Point Mutations Involved in Decreased Susceptibility to Macrolides, Lincosamides, Tetracyclines, and Spectinomycin. *Appl. Environ. Microbiol.* **2019**, *85*, e00575-19. [CrossRef] [PubMed]
35. Heuvelink, A.; Reugebrink, C.; Mars, J. Antimicrobial susceptibility of *Mycoplasma bovis* isolates from veal calves and dairy cattle in the Netherlands. *Vet. Microbiol.* **2016**, *189*, 1–7. [CrossRef] [PubMed]
36. Klein, U.; de Jong, A.; Youala, M.; El Garch, F.; Stevenin, C.; Moyaert, H.; Rose, M.; Catania, S.; Gyuranecz, M.; Pridmore, A.; et al. New antimicrobial susceptibility data from monitoring of *Mycoplasma bovis* isolated in Europe. *Vet. Microbiol.* **2019**, *238*, 108432. [CrossRef]
37. Lysnyansky, I.; Ayling, R.D. *Mycoplasma bovis*: Mechanisms of resistance and trends in antimicrobial susceptibility. *Front. Microbiol.* **2016**, 7. [CrossRef]
38. Sulyok, K.M.; Kreizinger, Z.; Fekete, L.; Hrivnak, V.; Magyar, T.; Janosi, S.; Schweitzer, N.; Turcsanyi, I.; Makrai, L.; Erdelyi, K.; et al. Antibiotic susceptibility profiles of *Mycoplasma bovis* strains isolated from cattle in Hungary, Central Europe. *BMC Vet. Res.* **2014**, *10*, 256. [CrossRef]
39. Jelinski, M.; Kinnear, A.; Gesy, K.; Andrés-Lasheras, S.; Zaheer, R.; Weese, S.; McAllister, A.T. Antimicrobial Sensitivity Testing of *Mycoplasma bovis* Isolates Derived from Western Canadian Feedlot Cattle. *Microorganisms* **2020**, *8*, 124. [CrossRef]
40. Anholt, R.M.; Klima, C.; Allan, N.; Matheson-Bird, H.; Schatz, C.; Ajitkumar, P.; Otto, S.J.; Peters, D.; Schmid, K.; Olson, M.; et al. Antimicrobial Susceptibility of Bacteria That Cause Bovine Respiratory Disease Complex in Alberta, Canada. *Front. Vet. Sci.* **2017**, 4. [CrossRef]
41. Klein, U.; de Jong, A.; Moyaert, H.; El Garch, F.; Leon, R.; Richard-Mazet, A.; Rose, M.; Maes, D.; Pridmore, A.; Thomson, J.R.; et al. Antimicrobial susceptibility monitoring of *Mycoplasma hyopneumoniae* and *Mycoplasma bovis* isolated in Europe. *Vet. Microbiol.* **2017**, *204*, 188–193. [CrossRef]
42. Woolums, A.R.; Karisch, B.B.; Frye, J.G.; Epperson, W.; Smith, D.R.; Blanton, J.; Austin, F.; Kaplan, R.; Hiott, L.; Woodley, T.; et al. Multidrug resistant *Mannheimia haemolytica* isolated from high-risk beef stocker cattle after antimicrobial metaphylaxis and treatment for bovine respiratory disease. *Vet. Microbiol.* **2018**, *221*, 143–152. [CrossRef]
43. Van Driessche, L.; Valgaeren, B.R.; Gille, L.; Boyen, F.; Ducatelle, R.; Haesebrouck, F.; Deprez, P.; Pardon, B. A Deep Nasopharyngeal Swab Versus Nonendoscopic Bronchoalveolar Lavage for Isolation of Bacterial Pathogens from Preweaned Calves With Respiratory Disease. *J. Vet. Intern. Med.* **2017**, *31*, 946–953. [CrossRef] [PubMed]
44. Vilei, E.M.; Bonvin-Klotz, L.; Zimmermann, L.; Ryser-Degiorgis, M.P.; Giacometti, M.; Frey, J. Validation and diagnostic efficacy of a TaqMan real-time PCR for the detection of *Mycoplasma conjunctivae* in the eyes of infected Caprinae. *J. Microbiol. Methods* **2007**, *70*, 384–386. [CrossRef] [PubMed]

45. Wisselink, H.J.; Smid, B.; Plater, J.; Ridley, A.; Andersson, A.M.; Aspan, A.; Pohjanvirta, T.; Vahanikkila, N.; Larsen, H.; Hogberg, J.; et al. A European interlaboratory trial to evaluate the performance of different PCR methods for *Mycoplasma bovis* diagnosis. *BMC Vet. Res.* **2019**, *15*, 12. [CrossRef] [PubMed]
46. Poumarat, F.; Longchambon, D.; Martel, J.L. Application of dot immunobinding on membrane filtration (MF dot) to the study of relationships within "*M. mycoides* cluster" and within "glucose and arginine-negative cluster" of ruminant mycoplasmas. *Vet. Microbiol.* **1992**, *32*, 375–390. [CrossRef]
47. Shimizu, T. Selective medium for the isolation of *Mycoplasma bovis* from nasal discharges of pneumonic calves. *Res. Vet. Sci.* **1983**, *34*, 371–373. [CrossRef]
48. Poumarat, F.; Perrin, B.; Longchambon, D. Identification of ruminant mycoplasmas by dot immunobinding on membrane filtration (MF dot). *Vet. Microbiol.* **1991**, *29*, 329–338. [CrossRef]

pathogens

MDPI

Article

Mycoplasma bovis in Spanish Cattle Herds: Two Groups of Multiresistant Isolates Predominate, with One Remaining Susceptible to Fluoroquinolones

Ana García-Galán [1], Laurent-Xavier Nouvel [2], Eric Baranowski [2], Ángel Gómez-Martín [1,3], Antonio Sánchez [1], Christine Citti [2] and Christian de la Fe [1,*]

1 Ruminant Health Research Group, Department of Animal Health, Faculty of Veterinary Sciences, Regional Campus of International Excellence "*Campus Mare Nostrum*", University of Murcia, 30100 Murcia, Spain; ana.garcia25@um.es (A.G.-G.); angel.gomezmartin@uchceu.es (A.G.-M.); asanlope@um.es (A.S.)

2 IHAP, ENVT, INRAE, Université de Toulouse, 31300 Toulouse, France; xavier.nouvel@envt.fr (L.-X.N.); eric.baranowski@envt.fr (E.B.); christine.citti@envt.fr (C.C.)

3 Microbiological Agents associated with Reproduction (*ProVaginBio*) Research Group, Department of Animal Health and Public Health, Faculty of Veterinary Sciences, University CEU Cardenal Herrera of Valencia, CEU Universities, 46113 Valencia, Spain

* Correspondence: cdelafe@um.es; Tel.: +34-868-88-72-59

Received: 5 June 2020; Accepted: 30 June 2020; Published: 7 July 2020

Abstract: *Mycoplasma bovis* is an important bovine pathogen causing pneumonia, mastitis, and arthritis and is responsible for major economic losses worldwide. In the absence of an efficient vaccine, control of *M. bovis* infections mainly relies on antimicrobial treatments, but resistance is reported in an increasing number of countries. To address the situation in Spain, *M. bovis* was searched in 436 samples collected from beef and dairy cattle (2016–2019) and 28% were positive. Single-locus typing using *polC* sequences further revealed that two subtypes ST2 and ST3, circulate in Spain both in beef and dairy cattle, regardless of the regions or the clinical signs. Monitoring of ST2 and ST3 isolates minimum inhibitory concentration (MIC) to a panel of antimicrobials revealed one major difference when using fluoroquinolones (FQL): ST2 is more susceptible than ST3. Accordingly, whole-genome sequencing (WGS) further identified mutations in the *gyrA* and *parC* regions, encoding quinolone resistance-determining regions (QRDR) only in ST3 isolates. This situation shows the capacity of ST3 to accumulate mutations in QRDR and might reflect the selective pressure imposed by the extensive use of these antimicrobials. MIC values and detection of mutations by WGS also showed that most Spanish isolates are resistant to macrolides, lincosamides, and tetracyclines. Valnemulin was the only one effective, at least in vitro, against both STs.

Keywords: *Mycoplasma bovis*; minimum inhibitory concentration; antimicrobial resistance; mutations; Spain

1. Introduction

Isolated in the early 60s, *Mycoplasma bovis* is an important bovine pathogen that has a major economic impact on the global cattle industry [1,2]. *M. bovis* is usually associated with a variety of clinical manifestations, including pneumonia, mastitis, arthritis, keratoconjunctivitis, otitis media, and genital disorders [2,3]. In the absence of an efficient vaccine, the control of *M. bovis* infections mainly relies on antimicrobial treatments [4]. However, many countries have reported that the in vitro antimicrobial sensitivity of *M. bovis* isolates has been dramatically reduced [5–14].

M. bovis belongs to the class *Mollicutes*, a large group of wall-less bacteria with reduced genome and limited metabolic capacities, but a remarkable adaptive potential [15,16]. Treatment with ß-lactams, glycopeptides, cycloserines, or fosfomycin is ineffective against *Mollicutes* infections since they all target cell-wall synthesis [17,18]. Similarly, polymyxins and sulfonamides/trimethoprim, whose primary targets are respectively membrane lipopolysaccharides and folic acid, are not effective against these organisms [17,18]. Finally, *Mollicutes* are also resistant to rifampicin due to a natural mutation in the *rpoB* gene of the RNA polymerase β subunit, which prevents the antibiotic from binding to its target [19–21]. Antimicrobials active against *Mycoplasmas* include macrolides, lincosamides, tetracyclines, amphenicols, and pleuromutilins, which are all interfering with the synthesis of proteins, and fluoroquinolones (FLQ), which are DNA synthesis inhibitors [22].

General guidelines for antimicrobial testing of veterinary mycoplasmas are available, although no standard or interpretative breakpoint has been formally published [23]. Hence, current minimum inhibitory concentration (MIC) data are supported by molecular evidence of genetic mutations associated with antimicrobial resistance [22,24]. Hot spot mutations in 16S rRNA genes, *rrs3* and *rrs4*, are related to resistance against tetracyclines, while those in 23S rRNA genes, *rrl3* and *rrl4*, are associated with resistance to macrolides, lincosamides, phenicols, and pleuromutilins. Mutations in *rplD* and *rplV* genes encoding ribosomal proteins L4 and L22 and *rplC* gene encoding L3 are also linked to resistance against macrolides and pleuromutilins, respectively. Finally, FLQ resistance is mainly associated with mutations in the quinolone resistance-determining regions (QRDR) of *gyrA* and *gyrB* genes encoding DNA-gyrase, and in *parC* and *parE* genes encoding topoisomerase IV [22,24].

In Europe, *M. bovis* is particularly damaging to the beef industry due to its contribution towards the bovine respiratory disease complex (BRD) that affects calves raised in feedlots [25–27]. This pathogen often acts in co-infection with other viruses and bacteria, although it is the only etiological agent found in the chronic forms of the disease [28]. Regarding the dairy industry, sporadic *M. bovis* outbreaks have been notified in Austria, Denmark, Switzerland, and The Netherlands. Based on field data from the analysis of bulk tank milk, the prevalence of the infection in France and the UK is less than 1%, and that in Belgium and Greece it is 1.5% and 5.4%, respectively [29–36].

The beef and dairy industry is crucial to Spain, yet little is known about the epidemiological situation of *M. bovis* infections in this country. The antimicrobial susceptibility of *M. bovis* isolates was recently monitored in different European countries, including Spain [37,38]. However, these studies only considered isolates collected from young animals with respiratory disease and did not provide complete, epidemiological background information regarding the isolates.

The spread of *M. bovis* infection in animals, herds, regions, or countries is usually associated with animal movements and the introduction of asymptomatic carriers, which are occasionally shedding the pathogen in milk, nasal, or genital secretions [2,3]. Animal exchanges between farms are common in the Spanish beef industry, which also imports a large number of animals from other European countries, with France being the main supplier, followed by Ireland and Germany [39]. Animal movements between dairy farms are less common since the replacement of dairy cows is usually performed with animals born in the same herd. Nevertheless, when the replacement rate is not sufficient to maintain milk production levels, external animals may be introduced to the herd, especially in larger farms. Interestingly, a study showed that infected semen was also at the origin of *M. bovis* mastitis outbreaks in two closed dairy herds in Finland [40].

Recently, a large molecular study, including *M. bovis* strains isolated in France from 1977 to 2012, revealed that two groups emerged after 2000 [41]. Based on their partial *polC* sequences, these corresponded to subtypes (STs) 2 and 3. Another study further observed a difference between the two STs in their ability to acquire FLQ resistance in vitro. While ST3 isolates are more likely to acquire mutations in their QRDR and become resistant under selective pressure, the genetic context of ST2 isolates appears to hinder the development of resistance [42]. Field isolates from both STs were found to be resistant to the macrolides tylosin and tilmicosin and the tetracycline, oxytetracycline, regardless of the associated clinical signs (respiratory disease, mastitis, otitis, or arthritis) [43]. Interestingly, the first multiresistant ST3 isolate reported in France was collected in 2011 from a calf born in Spain and raised in a veal-calf herd in Southwest France [41]. This raised the question of how the two STs were distributed in Spanish herds when considering a large number of field isolates, and whether their antimicrobial susceptibility profiles were congruent with *polC* typing. Spain, which allowed unrestricted use of FLQ until very recently, may serve as a clear in vivo model to study the effects of the indiscriminate use of these antimicrobials.

The present study objectives were (i) to assess the circulation of *M. bovis* in Spanish cattle herds using a large collection of isolates collected from beef and dairy cattle and from different sample sources (nasal, auricular, conjunctival, synovial fluid and tissues swabs, and mastitic milk); (ii) to subtype this collection by single-locus sequencing of *polC* [41]; (iii) to determine the antimicrobial susceptibility of *M. bovis* isolates studying differences between STs, with a focus on antimicrobial agents approved to treat bovine respiratory disease and/or mastitis in Spain; and (iv) to assess the occurrence of genetic mutations conferring antimicrobial resistance in a selection of isolates representative of each ST.

2. Results

2.1. *M. bovis Circulating in Spanish Beef and Dairy Herds Belongs to STs 2 and 3*

In this study, 93 (35.7%) of the 260 analyzed animals were infected with *M. bovis*. Among the 436 analyzed samples, a total of 165 tested positive for *Mycoplasma* spp. and *M. bovis* was the most commonly found species, with 122 PCR-positive samples.

Among beef cattle, *M. bovis* was detected in 84 (40.9%) of the 205 analyzed animals. Specifically, the pathogen was detected in 81 (44.3%) of the 183 feedlots calves and 3 (13.6%) of the 22 pasture-raised animals. The pathogen was detected in 40 (32%) of the 125 healthy animals and 44 (55%) of the 80 animals with clinical signs of respiratory disease or arthritis. Within the 331 analyzed samples, 102 were tested positive. Most positive samples were obtained from nasal swabs (85/278) and the remaining were identified in auricular swabs (5/27) and tissues swabs from lung (9/16), spleen (1/1), liver (1/2), and mediastinal lymph nodes (1/1). However, the pathogen was not found in conjunctival swabs (n = 3) nor synovial fluid (n = 3). The positive samples were obtained from 26 of the 30 analyzed farms and 5 of the 8 analyzed regions (Figure S1). Among dairy cattle, *M. bovis* was detected in 9 (16.36%) of the 55 analyzed animals. Specifically, the pathogen was detected in 9 (23.1%) of the 39 dairy cows with mastitis but was not detected in any of the 5 dairy calves with clinical signs of respiratory disease nor any of the 11 asymptomatic calves. Within the 105 analyzed samples, positive samples were only detected in mastitic milk (20/66), while any positive results were detected in BTM (n = 9), or nasal (n = 27), auricular (n = 1), or conjunctival (n = 2) swabs. The positive samples were obtained from 2 of the 7 farms and the milk analysis laboratory, and 3 of the 5 analyzed regions (Figure S1).

Globally, *M. bovis* was successfully isolated from 112 PCR-positive samples. Based on their origin, 95 representative isolates were chosen for further characterization (epidemiological background provided in Table S1 and illustrated in Figure 1). Briefly, the collection included isolates from beef (n = 75) and dairy cattle (n = 20). Beef cattle isolates were obtained from nasal (62/75), auricular (6/75), lung (6/75) and spleen swabs (1/75), asymptomatic (35/75) or with clinical signs of respiratory disease (33/75), arthritis (6/75), or both (1/75). Dairy cattle isolates were obtained from mastitic milk. Single-locus sequence analysis of *polC* revealed two ST profiles: ST2 (n = 37) and ST3 (n = 58). Both STs were found in beef and dairy cattle, in healthy or diseased animals and in different sample sources. Both STs were found concomitantly in animals from the same farm, or even in different samples from the same animal (Figure 1, Table S1). For example, isolates J96 and J102 (ST3) and J103 (ST2) were collected from spleen, nasal, and lung swabs of the same animal respectively (Table S1). Sequences corresponding to ST2 and ST3 are provided in Table S2.

Hence, no other STs than ST2 or ST3 were found in Spanish herds. Both STs were present in asymptomatic beef cattle or with clinical signs of respiratory disease or arthritis and in dairy cows with mastitis.

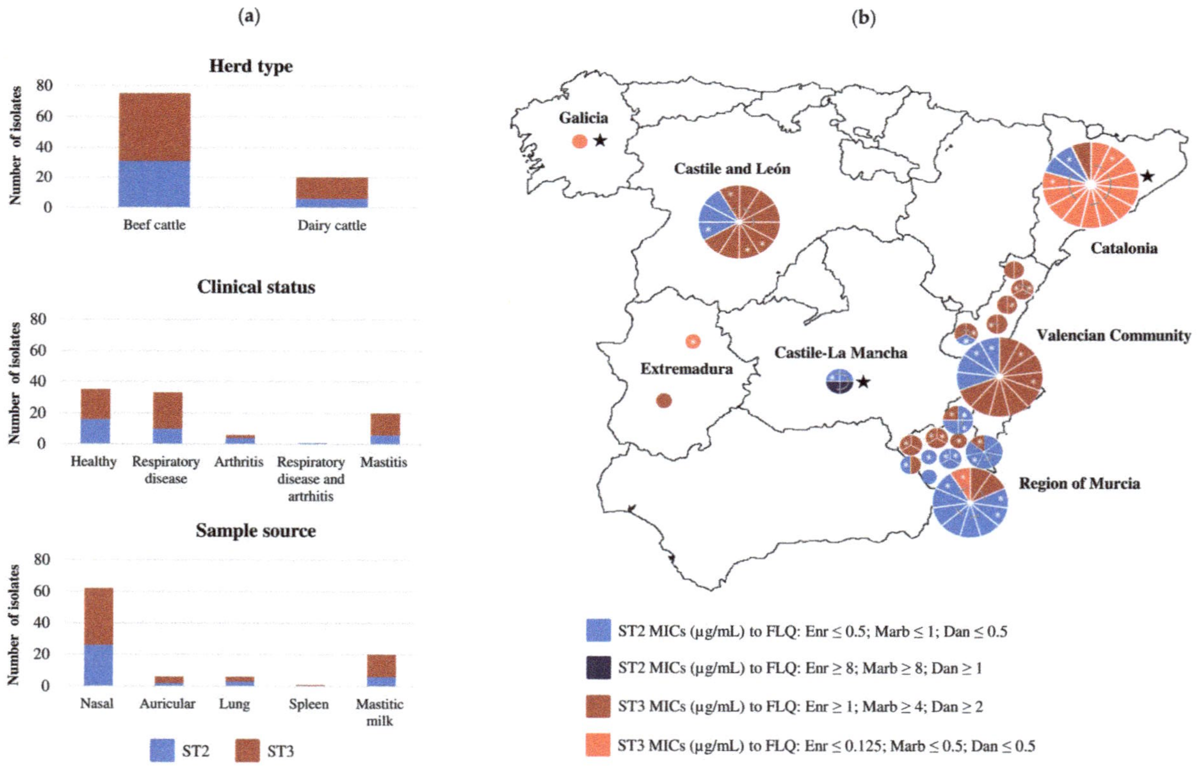

Figure 1. Epidemiological background of the 95 *Mycoplasma bovis* isolates included in this study: (**a**) Number of isolates of each subtype (ST) depending on the herd type, clinical status, and sample source; (**b**) Geographical origin of each isolate. Each circle represents a farm except in Catalonia, where a milk analysis laboratory provided samples. The radius of each circle is proportional to the number of isolates collected from the farm. Isolates collected from mastitic milk are indicated with a black star. Isolates linked with a grey line were obtained from the same animal. Isolates selected for whole-genome sequencing are indicated with a white asterisk. Enr = Enrofloxacin; Marb = Marbofloxacin; Dan = Danofloxacin.

2.2. The Antimicrobial Susceptibility Profiles of The Spanish Isolates to FLQ Differ Between PolC ST2 and ST3

The MIC values for the reference strain PG45 are shown in Table 1. Individual MIC values for each isolate are listed in Table S1. Statistical analyses revealed a significant difference in antimicrobial susceptibility to FLQ between ST2 and ST3 isolates ($p < 0.01$). No significant changes between STs were observed for macrolides, lincomycin, doxycycline, or valnemulin. The antimicrobial susceptibility profile of these two STs is illustrated in Table 1, Figures 1 and 2.

MIC values indicated a global decrease of *M. bovis* susceptibility to macrolides and lincomycin (MIC_{90} > 128), and to a lesser extent, doxycycline (MIC_{90} = 4 µg/mL). The majority of ST2 isolates (35/37) had low MIC values for FLQ (≤0.5 µg/mL for enrofloxacin and danofloxacin, and ≤ 1 µg/mL for marbofloxacin) (Figure 1, Table S1). Among the few exceptions were the isolates J320 and J323, obtained from mastitic milk of the same cow. The MIC of J320 was 16 µg/mL for enrofloxacin and marbofloxacin, and 1 µg/mL for danofloxacin and the MIC of J323 was 8 µg/mL for enrofloxacin and marbofloxacin, and 2 µg/mL for danofloxacin (Table S1). Interestingly, 4 ST2 isolates with different MIC profiles were obtained from the cranial quarters of that cow in different days: the isolates J319 (low MIC, left side) and J320 (high MIC, right side) one day, and the isolates J323 (high MIC, left side) and J324 (low MIC, right side) two days later (Figure 1, Table S1). On the contrary, most ST3 (43/58) isolates had high MIC values for FLQ (≥1, ≥4, and ≥2 µg/mL for enrofloxacin, marbofloxacin, and danofloxacin respectively). The remaining ST3 isolates (15/58) were collected from dairy cows with mastitis (13/15) and a few (2/15) from beef cattle with arthritis or asymptomatic (MIC ≤ 0.125 µg/mL for enrofloxacin, and ≤0.5 µg/mL for marbofloxacin and danofloxacin (Figure 1, Table S1). Finally, valnemulin was the only molecule that demonstrated activity against both STs.

Therefore, most of the *M. bovis* Spanish field isolates have a similar antimicrobial susceptibility profile against macrolides, lincomycin, and doxycycline with high MIC values and for valnemulin with low MIC values. On the contrary, antimicrobial susceptibility profiles against FLQ differed between ST2 and ST3, with high MIC values mainly associated with ST3 (Table 1).

Table 1. Minimum inhibitory concentration (MIC) ranges, MIC_{50} and MIC_{90} of *Mycoplasma bovis* isolates.

polC [a] ST	MIC Parameter	Macrolides			Lincosamide	Fluoroquinolones			Tetracycline	Pleuromutilin
		Tul	Gam	Tild	Lin	Enr	Marb	Dan	Dox	Val
1 PG45	MIC	1	8	1	1	0.125	0.5	0.125	0.0625	0.025
2 (n = 37)	MIC Range	16–>128	>128	>128	1–>128	0.125–16	0.25–16	0.125–2	0.25–4	0.025–0.2
	MIC_{50}	>128	>128	>128	>128	0.25	0.5	0.25	2	0.1
	MIC_{90}	>128	>128	>128	>128	0.5	1	0.5	4	0.1
3 (n = 58)	MIC Range	8–>128	>128	>128	1–>128	<0.0625–32	0.125–64	0.125–8	0.5–8	0.025–0.2
	MIC_{50}	>128	>128	>128	>128	16	32	4	2	0.1
	MIC_{90}	>128	>128	>128	>128	32	64	8	4	0.2

MIC values are given in µg/mL. Values are presented separately for each subtype (ST). The reference strain PG45 was used as control. Tul = Tulathromycin; Gam = Gamithromycin; Tild = Tildipirosin; Lin = Lincomycin; Enr = Enrofloxacin; Marb = Marbofloxacin; Dan = Danofloxacin; Dox = Doxycycline; Val = Valnemulin. [a] ST based on the single-locus sequence analysis of a region of the gene *polC* [41].

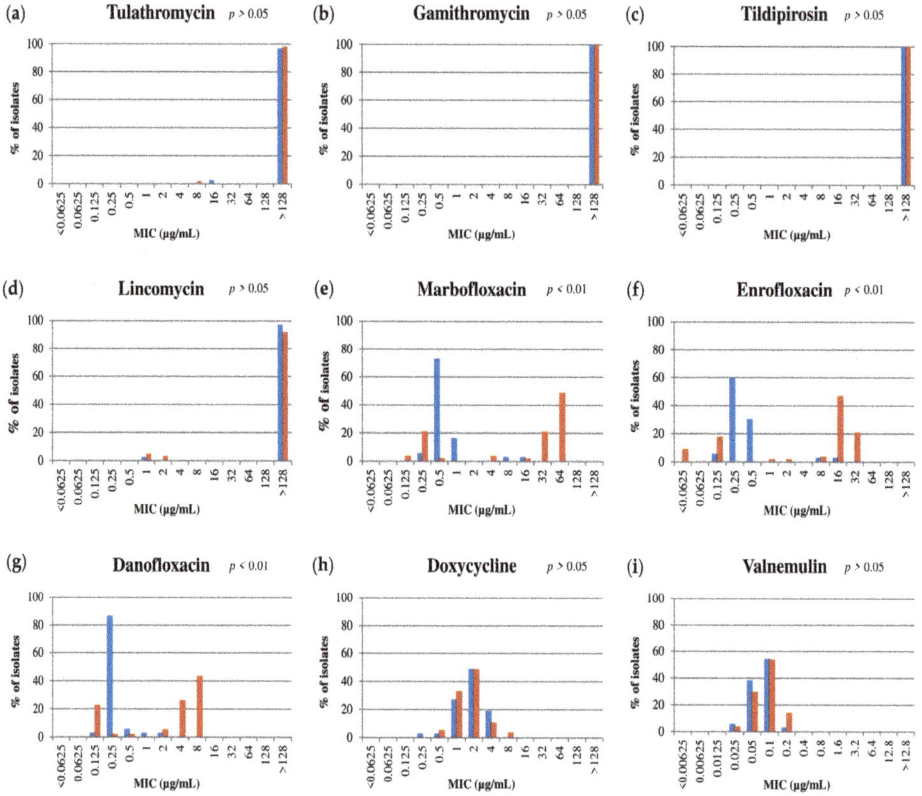

Figure 2. Minimum inhibitory concentration (MIC) distribution (%) of the 95 *Mycoplasma bovis* isolates for each antimicrobial included in this study: (**a**) Tulathromycin; (**b**) Gamithromycin; (**c**) Tildipirosin; (**d**) Lincomycin; (**e**) Marbofloxacin; (**f**) Enrofloxacin; (**g**) Danofloxacin; (**h**) Doxycycline; (**i**) Valnemulin. Blue bars correspond to subtype (ST) 2 and red bars to ST3. *P* values were obtained by comparing the log2MIC means between STs.

2.3. Analysis of Point Mutations Conferring Resistance to Antimicrobials: The Main Differences between ST2 and ST3 Are Found in The QRDR of GyrA and ParC Genes

A total of 36 *M. bovis* isolates belonging to ST2 (n = 16) and ST3 (n = 20) were subjected to whole-genome sequencing to compare nucleotide changes at QRDR, and rRNA (16S and 23S) and protein (L3, L4, and L22) genes (Tables 2–4). The epidemiological background of these isolates is provided in Table S1 and illustrated in Figure 1.

Nucleotide changes at QRDR revealed important differences between each ST, mainly located in *gyrA* and *parC*. While sequence analysis did not reveal any non-synonymous mutations in *gyrA* or *parC* for ST2 isolates, ST3 isolates were all characterized by at least one non-synonymous mutation in one or both genes. ST3 isolates were all characterized by a *parC* non-synonymous mutation at codon 10 (Gln10Arg). This mutation was associated with a substitution from serine to phenylalanine at *gyrA* codon 83 (Ser83Phe) and serine to isoleucine at *parC* codon 80 (Ser80Ile) in isolates with MIC values ≥ 1 µg/mL for FLQ. Among the few exceptions were the isolates J28, J228, and J279 having no mutation at *parC* codon 80, but a non-synonymous mutation at codon 116 (Ala116Pro in J228 and J279) or codons 81 and 84 (Ser81Pro; Asp84Asn in J28). Interestingly, while most of the ST2 and ST3 isolates showed a *gyrB* non-synonymous mutation associated with a substitution Asp362Asn, ST3 isolates J479, and J482 (MIC values ≥ 8 µg/mL for FLQ) were characterized by a substitution at *gyrB* codon 323

(Val323Ala) in combination with mutations Ser83Phe in *gyrA*, and Gln10Arg, Ser80Ile, and Val156Ile in *parC*.

Table 2. List of point mutations in the *gyrA*, *gyrB*, and *parC* quinolone resistance-determining regions (QRDR) identified in *Mycoplasma bovis* isolates and associated minimum inhibitory concentration (MIC) values for fluoroquinolones (FLQ).

Isolate	*polC* [a] ST	*gyrA*	*gyrB*		*parC*						MIC (μg/mL) [b]		
		83 [c]	362	323	10	80 [c]	81 [c]	84 [c]	116	156	Enr	Marb	Dan
PG45	1	Ser	Asp	Val	Gln	Ser	Ser	Asp	Ala	Val	0.125	0.5	0.125
J335	3	-	Asn	-	Arg	-	-	-	-	-	<0.0625	0.25	0.125
J403	3	-	Asn	-	Arg	-	-	-	-	-	<0.0625	0.25	0.125
J414	3	-	Asn	-	Arg	-	-	-	-	-	<0.0625	0.25	0.125
J433	3	-	Asn	-	Arg	-	-	-	-	-	0.125	0.25	0.125
J341	2	-	Asn	-	-	-	-	-	-	-	0.125	0.25	0.25
J6	2	-	Asn	-	-	-	-	-	-	-	0.25	0.5	0.25
J103	2	-	Asn	-	-	-	-	-	-	-	0.25	0.5	0.25
J175	2	-	Asn	-	-	-	-	-	-	-	0.25	0.5	0.25
J226	2	-	Asn	-	-	-	-	-	-	-	0.25	0.5	0.25
J276	2	-	Asn	-	-	-	-	-	-	-	0.25	0.5	0.25
J319	2	-	Asn	-	-	-	-	-	-	-	0.25	0.5	0.25
J330	2	-	Asn	-	-	-	-	-	-	-	0.25	0.5	0.25
J336	2	-	Asn	-	-	-	-	-	-	-	0.25	0.5	0.5
J356	2	-	Asn	-	-	-	-	-	-	-	0.25	0.5	0.25
J136	2	-	Asn	-	-	-	-	-	-	-	0.5	1	0.25
J137	2	-	Asn	-	-	-	-	-	-	-	0.5	0.5	0.125
J368	2	-	Asn	-	-	-	-	-	-	-	0.5	1	0.25
J377	2	-	Asn	-	-	-	-	-	-	-	0.5	1	0.25
J391	2	-	Asn	-	-	-	-	-	-	-	0.5	0.5	0.25
J410	2	-	Asn	-	-	-	-	-	-	-	0.5	0.5	0.25
J279	3	Phe	Asn	-	Arg	-	-	-	Pro	-	1	4	4
J228	3	Phe	Asn	-	Arg	-	-	-	Pro	-	2	4	2
J115	3	Phe	Asn	-	Arg	Ile	-	-	-	-	8	32	2
J28	3	Phe	Asn	-	Arg	-	Pro	Asn	-	-	16	64	8
J69	3	Phe	Asn	-	Arg	Ile	-	-	-	-	16	32	4
J72	3	Phe	Asn	-	Arg	Ile	-	-	-	-	16	64	8
J81	3	Phe	Asn	-	Arg	Ile	-	-	-	-	16	32	4
J96	3	Phe	Asn	-	Arg	Ile	-	-	-	-	16	32	4
J131	3	Phe	Asn	-	Arg	Ile	-	-	-	-	16	64	8
J305	3	Phe	Asn	-	Arg	Ile	-	-	-	-	16	64	8
J178	3	Phe	Asn	-	Arg	Ile	-	-	-	-	32	64	8
J233	3	Phe	Asn	-	Arg	Ile	-	-	-	-	32	64	8
J295	3	Phe	Asn	-	Arg	Ile	-	-	-	-	32	64	8
J388	3	Phe	Asn	-	Arg	Ile	-	-	-	-	32	64	8
J479	3	Phe	-	Ala	Arg	Ile	-	-	-	Ile	32	64	8
J482	3	Phe	-	Ala	Arg	Ile	-	-	-	Ile	32	64	8

Amino acid numbering refers to positions in *Escherichia coli* K12. [a] Subtype (ST) based on the single-locus sequence analysis of a region of the gene *polC* [41]. [b] Enr = Enrofloxacin; Marb = Marbofloxacin; Dan = Danofloxacin. [c] Mutations associated with FLQ resistance in previous studies [42,44–48].

Mutations in the 23S rRNA and 16S rRNA genes and the ribosomal proteins L3, L4, and L22 are listed in Table 3; Table 4. Regarding 23S rRNA, positions A534T, G748A were notably altered in both *rrl* alleles of all the isolates. Mutation A2058G affecting the majority of isolates (34/36) in one or both alleles was only absent in those with low MIC values for lincomycin (1 μg/mL). Mutations G954A in one or both alleles were altered in 31/36 isolates from both STs and the remaining five isolates had many compensatory non-synonymous mutations in L3, L4, and L22 proteins. Mutation T1249C in one allele was altered in 31/36 isolates from both STs. Mutations A1251T (1/36) and G2157A (5/36) in one allele and G2848T (2/36) in one allele were only found in ST3 isolates while G452A was present in one allele of a few number (5/36) of ST3 isolates. Some isolates from both STs (6/36) showed a single non-synonymous mutation in L4 or L22 (Table 3). Regarding 16S rRNA, mutations A965T and A967T were altered in both *rrs* alleles of all the isolates (MIC ≥ 1 μg/mL for doxycycline). Mutations C1192A in both alleles and T1199C in one or both alleles were altered in 31/36 isolates from both STs. Mutations C335T and C859T were present in one *rrs* allele of five isolates (from both STs) and one isolate (ST2) respectively (Table 4).

Hence, the main differences between ST2 and ST3 are found in the QRDR of *gyrA* and *parC* genes. None of the ST2 isolates have any amino acid substitution in either *gyrA* or *parC* while ST3 isolates with MIC values ≥ 1 μg/mL for FLQ have the mutation Ser83Phe in *gyrA* in combination with at least non-synonymous mutation in *parC* (positions 80, 81, 84, 116, and156).

Table 3. List of point mutations in 23S rRNA alleles of *Mycoplasma bovis* isolates and associated minimum inhibitory concentration (MIC) values for macrolides, lincomycin, and valnemulin.

Isolate	*polC* [a] ST	23S rRNA, *rrl* alleles [b]									L3 [c]	L4 [c]												L22 [c]		MIC (µg/mL) [d]				
		452	534	748 [e]	954	1249	1251	2058 [e,f]	2157	2848	265	11	24	36	44	62	63	68	79	94	178	178	178	5	93 [e]	Tul	Gam	Tild	Lin	Val
PG45	1	G	A	G	G	T	A	A	G	G	Ala	Ser	Thr	Thr	Ala	Val	Ala	Glu	Ala	Ala	Gly	Gly	Gly	Gln	Gln	1	8	1	1	0.025
J137	2	-	T **	A **	-	C *	-	-	-	-	Val	Thr	-	Ala	Thr	Ala	Thr	Ala	Thr	Thr	-	-	Val	-	His	16	>128	>128	1	0.1
J28	3	-	T **	A **	-	C *	-	-	-	-	Val	Thr	-	Ala	Thr	Ala	Thr	Ala	Thr	Thr	-	Leu	-	-	His	>128	>128	>128	1	0.05
J403	3	-	T **	A **	-	C *	-	G *	-	-	Val	Thr	-	-	Thr	Ala	Thr	Ala	Thr	Thr	Arg	-	-	-	His	>128	>128	>128	>128	0.1
J414	3	-	T **	A **	-	C *	-	G *	-	-	Val	Thr	-	Ala	Thr	Ala	Thr	Ala	Thr	Thr	Arg	-	-	-	His	>128	>128	>128	>128	0.1
J433	3	-	T **	A **	-	C *	-	G *	-	-	Val	Thr	-	Ala	Thr	Ala	Thr	Ala	Thr	Thr	Arg	-	-	-	His	>128	>128	>128	>128	0.1
J6	2	-	T **	A **	A *	C *	-	G **	-	-	-	-	-	-	-	-	-	-	-	-	-	-	-	-	-	>128	>128	>128	>128	0.1
J103	2	-	T **	A **	A *	C *	-	G **	-	-	-	-	Arg	-	-	-	-	-	-	-	-	-	-	-	-	>128	>128	>128	>128	0.025
J136	2	-	T **	A **	A *	C *	-	G **	-	-	-	-	-	-	-	-	-	-	-	-	-	-	-	Lys	-	>128	>128	>128	>128	0.05
J175	2	-	T **	A **	A *	C *	-	G **	-	-	-	-	-	-	-	-	-	-	-	-	-	-	-	-	-	>128	>128	>128	>128	0.05
J226	2	-	T **	A **	A *	C *	-	G **	-	-	-	-	-	-	-	-	-	-	-	-	-	-	-	-	-	>128	>128	>128	>128	0.1
J276	2	-	T **	A **	A *	C *	-	G **	-	-	-	-	-	-	-	-	-	-	-	-	-	-	-	-	-	>128	>128	>128	>128	0.05
J319	2	-	T **	A **	A *	C *	-	G **	-	-	-	-	-	-	-	-	-	-	-	-	-	-	-	-	-	>128	>128	>128	>128	0.05
J330	2	-	T **	A **	A *	C *	-	G **	-	-	-	-	-	-	-	-	-	-	-	-	-	-	-	-	-	>128	>128	>128	>128	0.1
J336	2	-	T **	A **	A *	C *	-	G **	-	-	-	-	-	-	-	-	-	-	-	-	-	-	-	-	-	>128	>128	>128	>128	0.05
J341	2	-	T **	A **	A *	C *	-	G **	-	-	-	-	-	-	-	-	-	-	-	-	-	-	-	-	-	>128	>128	>128	>128	0.05
J356	2	-	T **	A **	A *	C *	-	G **	-	-	-	-	-	-	-	-	-	-	-	-	-	-	-	-	-	>128	>128	>128	>128	0.1
J368	2	-	T **	A **	A *	C *	-	G **	-	-	-	-	-	-	-	-	-	-	-	-	-	-	-	-	-	>128	>128	>128	>128	0.1
J377	2	-	T **	A **	A *	C *	-	G **	-	-	-	-	-	-	-	-	-	-	-	-	-	-	-	-	-	>128	>128	>128	>128	0.05
J391	2	-	T **	A **	A *	C *	-	G **	-	-	-	-	-	-	-	-	-	-	-	-	-	-	-	-	-	>128	>128	>128	>128	0.2
J410	2	-	T **	A **	A *	C *	-	G **	-	-	-	-	-	-	-	-	-	-	-	-	-	-	-	-	-	>128	>128	>128	>128	0.1
J96	3	-	T **	A **	A *	C *	-	G **	A *	-	-	-	-	-	-	-	-	-	-	-	-	-	-	-	-	>128	>128	>128	>128	0.1
J178	3	-	T **	A **	A *	C *	-	G **	-	-	-	-	-	-	-	-	-	-	-	-	-	-	-	-	-	>128	>128	>128	>128	0.05
J228	3	-	T **	A **	A *	C *	-	G **	-	-	-	-	-	-	Thr	-	-	-	-	-	-	-	-	-	-	>128	>128	>128	>128	0.1
J233	3	-	T **	A **	A *	C *	-	G **	A *	-	-	-	-	-	-	-	-	-	-	-	-	-	-	-	-	>128	>128	>128	>128	0.1
J279	3	-	T **	A **	A *	C *	-	G **	-	-	-	-	-	-	-	-	-	-	-	-	-	-	-	-	-	>128	>128	>128	>128	0.1
J295	3	-	T **	A **	A *	C *	-	G **	A *	-	-	-	-	-	-	-	-	-	-	-	-	-	-	-	-	>128	>128	>128	>128	0.1

Table 3. *Cont.*

Isolate	*polC* [a] ST	23S rRNA, *rrl* alleles [b]									L3 [c]						L4 [c]							L22 [c]		MIC (μg/mL) [d]				
		452	534	748 [e]	954	1249	1251	2058 [e,f]	2157	2848	265	11	24	36	44	62	63	68	79	94	178	178	178	5	93 [e]	Tul	Gam	Tild	Lin	Val
J305	3	-	T **	A **	A *	C *	-	G **	A *	-	-	-	-	-	-	-	-	-	-	-	-	-	-	-	-	>128	>128	>128	>128	0.1
J335	3	-	T **	A **	A *	C *	T*	G **	-	-	-	-	-	-	-	-	-	-	-	-	-	-	-	-	-	>128	>128	>128	>128	0.05
J388	3	-	T **	A **	A *	C *	-	G **	A *	-	-	-	-	-	-	-	-	-	-	-	-	-	-	-	-	>128	>128	>128	>128	0.1
J479	3	-	T **	A **	A *	C *	-	G **	-	-	-	-	-	-	-	-	-	-	-	-	-	-	-	-	-	>128	>128	>128	>128	0.2
J482	3	-	T **	A **	A *	C *	-	G **	-	-	-	-	-	-	-	-	-	-	-	-	-	-	-	-	-	>128	>128	>128	>128	0.2
J69	3	A *	T **	A **	A **	-	-	G **	-	-	-	-	-	-	Thr	-	-	-	-	-	-	-	-	-	-	>128	>128	>128	>128	0.05
J72	3	A *	T **	A **	A **	-	-	G **	-	-	-	-	-	-	-	-	-	-	-	-	-	-	-	-	-	>128	>128	>128	>128	0.05
J81	3	A *	T **	A **	A **	-	-	G **	-	T *	-	-	-	-	-	-	-	-	-	-	-	-	-	-	-	>128	>128	>128	>128	0.1
J115	3	A *	T **	A **	A **	-	-	G **	-	T *	-	-	-	-	Thr	-	-	-	-	-	-	-	-	-	-	>128	>128	>128	>128	0.025
J131	3	A *	T **	A **	A **	-	-	G **	-	-	-	-	-	-	Thr	-	-	-	-	-	-	-	-	-	-	>128	>128	>128	>128	0.1

[a] Subtype (ST) based on the single-locus sequence analysis of a region of the gene *polC* [41]; [b] nucleotide numbering refers to *Escherichia coli* K12; a single * indicates mutation in one *rrl* allele and ** indicates mutation in both alleles; [c] amino acid numbering refers to positions in PG45; [d] Tul= Tulathromycin; Gam = Gamithromycin; Tild = Tildipirosin; Lin = Lincomycin; Val = Valnemulin. [e] Mutations associated with macrolides resistance in *M. bovis* [43,47,49]. [f] Mutation associated with lincomycin resistance in *Mycoplasma synoviae* [50].

Table 4. List of point mutations in 16S rRNA alleles of *Mycoplasma bovis* isolates and associated minimum inhibitory concentration (MIC) values for doxycycline.

Isolate	*polC* [a] ST	16S rRNA, *rrs* alleles [b]						MIC (µg/mL) [c]
		335	859	965 [d]	967 [d]	1192 [e]	1199	Dox
PG45	1	C	C	A	A	C	T	0.0625
J137	2	T *	T *	T **	T **	-	-	1
J28	3	T *	-	T **	T **	-	-	1
J403	3	T *	-	T **	T **	-	-	1
J414	3	T *	-	T **	T **	-	-	1
J433	3	T *	-	T **	T **	-	-	1
J276	2	-	-	T **	T **	A **	C **	1
J319	2	-	-	T **	T **	A **	C **	1
J341	2	-	-	T **	T **	A **	C **	1
J115	3	-	-	T **	T **	A **	C **	1
J335	3	-	-	T **	T **	A **	C **	1
J6	2	-	-	T **	T **	A **	C **	2
J103	2	-	-	T **	T **	A **	C **	2
J136	2	-	-	T **	T **	A **	C **	2
J175	2	-	-	T **	T **	A **	C **	2
J226	2	-	-	T **	T **	A **	C **	2
J336	2	-	-	T **	T **	A **	C **	2
J356	2	-	-	T **	T **	A **	C **	2
J377	2	-	-	T **	T **	A **	C **	2
J391	2	-	-	T **	T **	A **	C **	2
J410	2	-	-	T **	T **	A **	C **	2
J69	3	-	-	T **	T **	A **	C **	2
J72	3	-	-	T **	T **	A **	C **	2
J81	3	-	-	T **	T **	A **	C **	2
J178	3	-	-	T **	T **	A **	C **	2
J228	3	-	-	T **	T **	A **	C *	2
J279	3	-	-	T **	T **	A **	C *	2
J295	3	-	-	T **	T **	A **	C **	2
J305	3	-	-	T **	T **	A **	C **	2
J479	3	-	-	T **	T **	A **	C *	2
J482	3	-	-	T **	T **	A **	C *	2
J330	2	-	-	T **	T **	A **	C **	4
J368	2	-	-	T **	T **	A **	C **	4
J131	3	-	-	T **	T **	A **	C **	4
J233	3	-	-	T **	T **	A **	C **	4
J96	3	-	-	T **	T **	A **	C **	8
J388	3	-	-	T **	T **	A **	C **	8

[a] Subtype (ST) based on the single-locus sequence analysis of a region of the gene *polC* [41]; [b] nucleotide numbering refers to *Escherichia coli K12;* a single * indicates mutation in one *rrl* allele and ** indicates mutation in both alleles; [c] Dox = doxycycline. [d] Mutations associated with *M bovis* tetracyclines resistance in previous studies [43,51]. [e] Mutation associated with spectinomycin resistance in previous studies [47,48].

3. Discussion

M. bovis was found to be widely distributed in Spanish cattle herds. More specifically, *M. bovis* was mainly detected in feedlot calves (81/183) and to a lesser extent in pasture-raised animals (3/22) housed in 26 different farms from 5 Spanish regions. This pathogenic species was not only detected in animals suffering from respiratory infections and/or arthritis (44/80), but also in asymptomatic carriers (40/125). These results consolidate previous studies that reported the isolation of *M. bovis* from young cattle with respiratory disease in Spain between 2010–2012 and 2015–2016 [37,38]. Although the complete epidemiological background of those isolates was not provided, the authors indicated that each isolate was obtained from a different farm. Altogether, these data indicate that, at least among beef cattle, the infection may have already become endemic, as reported in other European countries [25–27]. The presence of asymptomatic carriers and the movement of cattle between beef cattle farms, which frequently involves the mix of animals of diverse origins [39], may explain the current situation in Spain. The isolation of *M. bovis* from clinical mastitis cases was unusual given the low prevalence of this infection in other European countries. Therefore, further studies are needed to confirm whether this particular situation only reflects a bias of the sampling procedure or indicates that Spain is facing an important increase in the number of mastitis cases associated with *M. bovis*.

M. bovis isolates circulating in Spain are divided into two *polC* STs, 2 and 3. These two STs are similar to recent French isolates [41–43]. Compared with France, where ST2 has been predominant since 2000 [41–43], almost two thirds (58/95) of the characterized Spanish isolates belong to ST3. Both STs are widely distributed among different farms and regions, and can be isolated from beef and dairy cattle, from animals with different clinical conditions, and even from different anatomic locations of the same animal. This argues in favor of an efficient circulation and transmission of both STs, as already suggested with French isolates. Thus, animal movement between farms, a common practice in the Spanish beef cattle industry, is likely contributing to the dissemination of *M. bovis* [39]. Animal movements between dairy farms is less common, but asymptomatic carriers can be introduced into the herd when the replacement rate of animals born in the same herd is insufficient to maintain milk production. Furthermore, artificial insemination may be another way of entry for *M. bovis*. This was recently documented in Finland, where semen was reported to be the source of *M. bovis* mastitis outbreaks in two dairy herds [40].

Antimicrobial susceptibility profiles against FLQ differed between ST2 and ST3 isolates. The analysis of the QRDR revealed that the main differences between these STs were located in *gyrA* and *parC*. Remarkably, ST3 isolates were all characterized by an unusual Gln10Arg mutation in *parC*. This mutation is unrelated to antimicrobial resistance, since it was found in ST3 isolates associated with high and low MIC values ($\geq$ 1 and $\leq$ 1 µg/mL, respectively), and are likely to reflect phylogenetic evolution. ST3 isolates with MIC values $\geq$ 1 µg/mL were all characterized by mutation Ser83Phe in *gyrA* in combination with one or more amino acid substitution (Ser80Ile, Ser81Pro, Asp84Asn, Ala116Pro, or Val156Ile) in *parC*. Only three of these *parC* mutations, Ser80Ile, Ser81Pro, andAsp84Asn, have been previously described [42,45–48]. A point mutation Ser83Phe in *GyrA* is sufficient to reach an intermediate level of susceptibility to FLQ but additional substitutions in *parC* are required for resistance [42,44–48]. Interestingly, ST2 and a majority of ST3 (18/20) isolates had the mutation Asp362Asn in *gyrB*. This mutation also appears in recent French isolates and is related to phylogenetic evolution rather than drug resistance [41,42]. Two ST3 isolates harbor a Val323Ala mutation in *gyrB*, but its contribution to FLQ resistance is unknown.

Our results are consistent with in vitro studies showing that under selective pressure, ST3 isolates are more prone to accumulate QRDR mutations than ST2 isolates. Therefore, the widespread circulation of FLQ-resistant ST3 isolates in Spain might reflect the overuse of these antimicrobials in the field. Remarkably, two ST2 isolates were also found to be resistant to FLQ. They were isolated from a cow with clinical mastitis together with susceptible ST2 isolates. This may be the result of long-term treatment with FLQ, leading to the generation of resistant strains, and re-infection with susceptible strains. Globally, our results contrast with other countries where most *M. bovis* strains are susceptible to this family of antimicrobials [6,9–13].

MIC values confirmed the general decrease of *M. bovis* susceptibility to macrolides and lincomycin (MIC_{90} > 128) [5,9–13]. Analysis of 23S rRNA genes revealed that isolates with MIC values > 128 µg/mL for macrolides and lincomycin acquired mutations G748A (in both *rrl* alleles) and A2058G (in one or both *rrl* alleles). A combination of mutations in these hotspots is necessary and sufficient to achieve resistance to other macrolides, such as tylosin and tilmicosin, while mutation A2058G in one or both alleles has been linked to lincomycin resistance in *M. synoviae* [43,49,50]. Isolates J28 and J137 showed high MIC values (16–128 μg/mL) for macrolides but did not carry the mutation A2058G. Consistently, they are the only isolates with low MIC values for lincomycin (1 μg/mL). However, both isolates have several non-synonymous mutations in L4 and L22 proteins including Gln93His in L22, which is related to macrolide resistance and could explain the observed high MIC values for these antimicrobials [43]. No other point mutations related to antimicrobial resistance have been found in the *rrl* alleles or in L4 and L22 proteins. Since they appear together with other mutations conferring resistance, it is difficult to determine their importance.

As expected by the in vitro antimicrobial activity of pleuromutilins against a broad range of veterinary mycoplasmas [22], valnemulin was the only antimicrobial that demonstrated activity against both STs. Indeed, no mutation previously associated with pleuromutilin resistance [47] has been observed in any isolate. This is consistent with the fact that pleuromutilins are only registered for treatment in swine and poultry [52]. Valnemulin may thus be an interesting therapeutic alternative as it has been shown to be effective for the treatment of calves experimentally infected with *M. bovis* [53].

Overall, low in vitro susceptibility was observed for doxycycline (MIC_{90} = 4 μg/mL). Analysis of 16S rRNA genes revealed that isolates with MIC values ≥ 1 μg/mL were characterized by mutations A965T and A967T in both *rrs* alleles. Previous studies have concluded that this double mutation causes decreased susceptibility to other antimicrobials from the same group, such as oxytetracycline and tetracycline [43,51]. Mutations C1192A and T1199C were previously described in French isolates [43], although they did not further modify MIC values as it occurs with Spanish isolates. However, the mutation C1192A has been described both in Hungarian and Japanese isolates and was associated with high MIC values for spectinomycin [47,48]. As expected, mutations C335T and C859T, which have never been associated with antimicrobial resistance, had no influence on the susceptibility of the Spanish isolates. Finally, our results were also consistent with data suggesting that after macrolides, the highest resistances of the main veterinary mycoplasmas species are observed for tetracyclines [22].

In conclusion, our study revealed the extended circulation of *M. bovis* in Spanish beef cattle herds and its implication in mastitis cases. Circulating isolates are divided into two groups, ST2 and ST3, both being resistant to macrolides, lincosamides and tetracyclines. Most ST3 isolates circulating in Spain are resistant to FLQ, a situation which illustrates the remarkable capacity of ST3 to accumulate mutations in QRDR and the selective pressure imposed by the indiscriminate use of these antimicrobials. Valnemulin has been shown to be very effective against both STs in vitro, and its effectiveness in vivo should be further investigated.

4. Materials and Methods

4.1. Animal Sampling

All animal procedures were performed following the EU Directive 2010/63/EU for animal experimentation and had the authorization of the Ethics Committee on Animal Testing of the University of Murcia (Number: 307/2017).

In this study, 260 animals from 10 Spanish regions were sampled over a 4 year period (2016–2019). A total of 433 samples were collected from beef and dairy cattle.

Among beef cattle, 183 calves were raised in feedlots and 22 pasture-raised animals were sampled. Healthy animals (n = 125) and animals with clinical symptoms of respiratory disease or arthritis (n = 80) were both considered. In total, 331 samples were obtained from beef cattle. The sample collection was composed of nasal swabs (n = 278), auricular (n = 27) and conjunctival swabs (n = 3), synovial fluid (n = 3), as well as a number of swabs from tissues (lung, n = 16; liver, n = 2; spleen, n = 1; and mediastinal lymph node, n = 1). Those samples were obtained from 30 farms and 8 different regions (Figure S1).

Among dairy cattle, 39 cows with mastitis, and 16 calves with clinical signs of respiratory disease (n = 5) or asymptomatic (n = 11) were sampled. In total, 105 samples were obtained from dairy cattle. The sample collection was composed of mastitic milk (n = 66), bulk tank milk (BTM) (n = 9), and nasal (n = 27), auricular (n = 1), and conjunctival swabs (n = 2). Those samples were obtained from 7 farms and a milk analyses laboratory that provided samples and they were taken from 5 different regions (Figure S1).

4.2. *Mycoplasma Isolation and Subtyping*

For mycoplasma isolation from animal samples, swabs or mastitic milk samples (200 μL) were incubated at 37 °C for 24 h in 2 mL of SP4 medium [54] with modifications (Appendix A). Cultures were filtered through a 0.45 μm membrane filter (LLG-Labware, UK) and further incubated for 48 h before plating 5 μL onto solid SP4 medium. Agar plates were grown at 37 °C and examined daily under the microscope for the presence of mycoplasma colonies with the typical fried egg morphology.

The DNA extraction was performed from 200 μL of culture [55]. *M. bovis* detection was performed by PCR amplification of the membrane protein 81 gene [56]. *M. bovis* PCR positive cultures were three times cloned by picking single colonies and the identity of the final isolate was confirmed again by PCR.

M. bovis subtyping was performed by sequence analysis of a 520 bp region of the *polC* gene, as previously described [41]. Amplicon sequencing was performed at the molecular biology service of the University of Murcia and sequence analyses were conducted using MEGA 6 [57].

4.3. *MIC Assays*

Antimicrobials used for MIC assays included (i) the macrolides, tulathromycin (Carbosiynth, Compton, UK), gamithromycin (Sigma-Aldrich, St. Louis, MO, USA) and tildipirosin (Carbosiynth, Compton, UK), (ii) the lincosamide, lincomycin (Sigma-Aldrich, St. Louis, MO, USA), (iii) the FLQ, enrofloxacin (Fluka, Bio-Chemika, St. Louis, MO, USA), marbofloxacin (Tokio Chemical Industry, Chuo City, Japan) and danofloxacin (Fluka, Bio-Chemika, St. Louis, MO, USA), (iv) the tetracycline, doxycycline (Sigma-Aldrich, St. Louis, MO, USA), and (v) the pleuromutilin, valnemulin hydrochloride (Sigma-Aldrich, St. Louis, MO, USA). Stock solutions (1 mg/mL; 0.1 mg/mL for valnemulin hydrochloride) and two-fold dilutions were prepared in sterile distilled water. For preparing enrofloxacin, marbofloxacin, and danofloxacin, 0.1 M HCl was added dropwise until dissolution occurred and the volume was adjusted with sterile distilled water. A final range from 128 μg/mL to 0.0625 μg/mL was tested except for valnemulin, for which a final range from 12.8 μg/mL to 0.00625 μg/mL was studied.

Stationary-phase cultures of 95 *M. bovis* isolates and the reference strain PG45 were used for MIC assays. Mycoplasma cultures were carried out in PH medium [58] without antimicrobials, supplemented with sodium pyruvate (0.5%) and phenol red (0.005%), and mycoplasma titers were determined as previously described [59]. MIC assays were carried out in 96-well microtiter plates using the microbroth dilution method [23]. Briefly, 25.6 μL of each antimicrobial dilution and 25 μL of the diluted *M. bovis* inoculum (10^3–10^5 CFU/mL) were added to 150 μL of culture medium. Additionally, a positive control (well without antimicrobial) and a negative control (well without neither antimicrobial nor inoculum) were included in each essay. After 48 h of incubation at 37 °C, plates were examined for color change. MIC was defined as the lowest concentration of antimicrobial capable of completely inhibiting the growth of *M. bovis*. For each antimicrobial, the MIC range, MIC_{50} (lowest concentration of antimicrobial capable of inhibiting the growth of 50% of the isolates), and MIC_{90} (lowest concentration of antimicrobial capable of inhibiting the growth of 90% of the isolates) were calculated. All the assays were performed in duplicate. For accepting the results, MIC values of the duplicate tests had to be within one dilution, with the higher MIC value being used. If not, a third assay was performed, and the final MIC value was the mode of the three values.

4.4. Statistical Analysis

MIC values were transformed to a continuous variable by calculating their Log2 values. Log2MIC means values of ST2 and ST3 isolates were compared for each antimicrobial. Statistical analyses were run using the EpiInfo software [60] using ANOVA or Mann–Whitney/Wilcoxon Two-Sample Test (Kruskal–Wallis test for two groups) according to the inequality of population variances and with the significance level set at 0.01.

4.5. Whole-Genome Sequencing

Genomic DNA was extracted from a selection of 36 isolates (Table S1) from 15 mL of mycoplasma culture using a High Pure PCR Template Preparation Kit (Roche, Bâle, Suisse) according to the manufacturer's instructions. Whole-genome sequencing was performed using Illumina technology Hiseq (paired-end, 2 × 150pb) by Novogene Europe (Cambridge, UK). Bioinformatics analyses were performed on Galaxy platform (Genotoul, Toulouse, France). Quality controls of reads were performed using *FastQC* tool [61]. Alignments were carried out with *BWA-MEM* using PG45 as the reference [62], and alignments quality controls were checked with *QualiMap BamQC* [63]. SNP identification was done by alignment visualization with *Integrative Genomics Viewer* (IGV 2.7.0) [64] or by variant calling analysis with *breseq* [65]. All sequence files are available from the European Nucleotide Archive database (ENA), under study accession number PRJEB38707.

Supplementary Materials: The following are available online at http://www.mdpi.com/2076-0817/9/7/545/s1, Figure S1: Map of Spain showing the autonomous communities (AC) and the origin of the samples, Table S1: Epidemiological background, *polC* characterization and minimum inhibitory concentration (MIC) values of the 95 *Mycoplasma bovis* isolates, Table S2: Partial sequences (520 pb) types of the *polC* gene.

Author Contributions: Conceptualization, L.-X.N., and C.d.l.F.; methodology, A.G.-G., L.-X.N., Á.G.-M., A.S., and C.d.l.F.; software, A.G.-G., L.-X.N., and A.S.; validation, A.G.-G., L.-X.N., A.S., and C.d.l.F.; formal analysis, A.G.-G., L.-X.N., and C.d.l.F.; investigation, A.G.-G., L.-X.N., E.B., and C.d.l.F.; resources, C.d.l.F.; data curation, A.G.-G., L.-X.N., and C.d.l.F.; writing—original draft preparation, A.G.-G., L.-X.N., and E.B.; writing—review and editing, A.G.-G., L.-X.N., E.B., C.C., and C.d.l.F.; visualization, A.G.-G., L.-X.N., E.B., Á.G.-M., A.S., C.C., and C.d.l.F.; supervision, L.-X.N., Á.G.-M., and C.d.l.F.; project administration, C.d.l.F.; funding acquisition, C.d.l.F. All authors have read and agreed to the published version of the manuscript.

Funding: This research has been supported by the Spanish Ministry of Economy and Competitiveness (Spanish Government) co-financed by FEDER funds, project AGL2016-76568-R. Ana García-Galán Pérez is a beneficiary of a research fellowship (State Subprogram Training of the State Program for the Promotion of Talent and its Employability, BES-2017-080186).

Acknowledgments: The authors are grateful to: Ángel García Muñoz, Juan Seva Alcaraz, and Juan Alcazar Triviño for providing us the contacts for taking samples; to Mercè Lazaro for providing us the mastitic milk samples received in her laboratory; to the veterinarians that collected samples in the field; to the farmers for allowing the collection of the samples; to the Genotoul bioinformatics platform Toulouse Midi-Pyrenees for providing help and storage resources.

Conflicts of Interest: The authors declare no conflict of interest. The funders had no role in the design of the study; in the collection, analyses, or interpretation of data; in the writing of the manuscript, or in the decision to publish the results.

Appendix A

The medium SP4 was prepared following previous recommendations [54] but with some modifications.The modified medium is composed of three parts (A, B, and C). Part A is composed of 4.2 g of Difco PPLO broth (BD), 6.4 g of Bacto Peptone (BD), 12 g of Bacto Tryptone (BD) and 724 mL of deionized water. The solid medium includes 7 g of European Bacteriological Agar (Conda-Pronadisa). The pH is adjusted to 7.8 and then part A is autoclaved at 121 °C for 20 min. Part B is composed of 60 mL of RPMI-1640 (Sigma-Aldrich), 21 mL of fresh yeast extract 50% *w*/*v*, 2.4 g of yeast extract (Conda-Pronadisa), 4.8 mL of phenol red 0.5%, (Sigma-Aldrich) and 0.642 g of ampicillin sodium salt (Fisher bioreagents). The pH is adjusted to 7.2 and then part B is filter-sterilized through a 0.2 μL pore size filter. Part C is composed of 251 mL of heat-inactivated horse serum (Hyclone) for 30 min at 56 °C.

References

1. Hale, H.H.; Helmboldt, C.F.; Plastridge, W.N.; Stula, E.F. Bovine mastitis caused by a Mycoplasma species. *Cornell Vet.* **1962**, *52*, 582–591. [PubMed]
2. Nicholas, R.A.J.; Ayling, R.D. *Mycoplasma bovis*: Disease, diagnosis, and control. *Res. Vet. Sci.* **2003**, *74*, 105–112. [CrossRef]
3. Maunsell, F.P.; Woolums, A.R.; Francoz, D.; Rosenbusch, R.F.; Step, D.L.; Wilson, D.J.; Janzen, E.D. *Mycoplasma bovis* infections in cattle. *J. Vet. Intern. Med.* **2011**, *25*, 772–783. [CrossRef] [PubMed]
4. Perez-Casal, J.; Prysliak, T.; Maina, T.; Suleman, M.; Jimbo, S. Status of the development of a vaccine against Mycoplasma bovis. *Vaccine* **2017**, *35*, 2902–2907. [CrossRef]
5. Gerchman, I.; Levisohn, S.; Mikula, I.; Lysnyansky, I. In vitro antimicrobial susceptibility of *Mycoplasma bovis* isolated in Israel from local and imported cattle. *Vet. Microbiol.* **2009**, *137*, 268–275. [CrossRef]
6. Soehnlen, M.K.; Kunze, M.E.; Karunathilake, K.E.; Henwood, B.M.; Kariyawasam, S.; Wolfgang, D.R.; Jayarao, B.M. In vitro antimicrobial inhibition of *Mycoplasma bovis* isolates submitted to the Pennsylvania Animal Diagnostic Laboratory using flow cytometry and a broth microdilution method. *J. Vet. Diagn.* **2011**, *23*, 547–551. [CrossRef]
7. Hendrick, S.H.; Bateman, K.G.; Rosengren, L.B. The effect of antimicrobial treatment and preventive strategies on bovine respiratory disease and genetic relatedness and antimicrobial resistance of *Mycoplasma bovis* isolates in a western Canadian feedlot. *Can. Vet. J. Rev. Vet. Can.* **2013**, *54*, 1146–1156.
8. Ayling, R.D.; Rosales, R.S.; Barden, G.; Gosney, F.L. Changes in antimicrobial susceptibility of *Mycoplasma bovis* isolates from Great Britain. *Vet. Rec.* **2014**, *175*, 486. [CrossRef]
9. Gautier-Bouchardon, A.V.; Ferré, S.; Le Grand, D.; Paoli, A.; Gay, E.; Poumarat, F. Overall decrease in the susceptibility of *Mycoplasma bovis* to antimicrobials over the past 30 years in France. *PLoS ONE* **2014**, *9*, e87672. [CrossRef]
10. Kawai, K.; Higuchi, H.; Iwano, H.; Iwakuma, A.; Onda, K.; Sato, R.; Hayashi, T.; Nagahata, H.; Oshida, T. Antimicrobial susceptibilities of Mycoplasma isolated from bovine mastitis in Japan. *Anim. Sci. J.* **2014**, *85*, 96–99. [CrossRef]
11. Sulyok, K.M.; Kreizinger, Z.; Fekete, L.; Hrivnák, V.; Magyar, T.; Jánosi, S.; Schweitzer, N.; Turcsányi, I.; Makrai, L.; Erdélyi, K.; et al. Antibiotic susceptibility profiles of *Mycoplasma bovis* strains isolated from cattle in Hungary, Central Europe. *BMC Vet. Res.* **2014**, *10*, 256. [CrossRef] [PubMed]
12. Heuvelink, A.; Reugebrink, C.; Mars, J. Antimicrobial susceptibility of *Mycoplasma bovis* isolates from veal calves and dairy cattle in the Netherlands. *Vet. Microbiol.* **2016**, *189*, 1–7. [CrossRef] [PubMed]
13. Kong, L.C.; Gao, D.; Jia, B.Y.; Wang, Z.; Gao, Y.-H.; Pei, Z.-H.; Liu, S.-M.; Xin, J.-Q.; Ma, H.-X. Antimicrobial susceptibility and molecular characterization of macrolide resistance of *Mycoplasma bovis* isolates from multiple provinces in China. *J. Vet. Med. Sci.* **2016**, *78*, 293–296. [CrossRef]
14. Jelinski, M.; Kinnear, A.; Gesy, K.; Andrés-Lasheras, S.; Zaheer, R.; Weese, S.; McAllister, T.A. Antimicrobial sensitivity testing of *Mycoplasma bovis* isolates derived from Western Canadian feedlot cattle. *Microorganisms* **2020**, *8*, 124. [CrossRef]
15. Citti, C.; Dordet-Frisoni, E.; Nouvel, L.X.; Kuo, C.; Baranowski, E. Horizontal gene transfers in mycoplasmas (Mollicutes). *Curr. Issues Mol. Biol.* **2018**, 3–22. [CrossRef] [PubMed]
16. Faucher, M.; Nouvel, L.-X.; Dordet-Frisoni, E.; Sagné, E.; Baranowski, E.; Hygonenq, M.-C.; Marenda, M.-S.; Tardy, F.; Citti, C. Mycoplasmas under experimental antimicrobial selection: The unpredicted contribution of horizontal chromosomal transfer. *PLoS Genet.* **2019**, *15*, e1007910. [CrossRef]
17. McCormack, W.M. Susceptibility of mycoplasmas to antimicrobial agents: Clinical implications. *Clin. Infect. Dis.* **1993**, *17* (Suppl. S1), S200–S201. [CrossRef] [PubMed]
18. Olaitan, A.O.; Morand, S.; Rolain, J.M. Mechanisms of polymyxin resistance: Acquired and intrinsic resistance in bacteria. *Front. Microbiol.* **2014**, *5*, 643. [CrossRef] [PubMed]
19. Gadeau, A.P.; Mouches, C.; Bove, J.M. Probable insensitivity of mollicutes to rifampin and characterization of spiroplasmal DNA-dependent RNA polymerase. *J. Bacteriol.* **1986**, *166*, 824–828. [CrossRef]
20. Pellegrin, J.L.; Maugein, J.; Clerc, M.T.; Leng, B.; Bové, J.M.; Bébéar, C. Activity of rifampin against Mollicutes, clostridia and L forms. Recent advances in mycoplasmology. *Zentralbl. Bakteriol. Suppl.* **1990**, *20*, 810–812.

21. Shepard, M.C.; Lunceford, C.D.; Ford, D.K.; Purcell, R.H.; Taylor-Robinson, D.; Razin, S.; Black, F.T. Ureaplasma urealyticum gen. nov., sp. nov.: Proposed nomenclature for the human T (T-Strain) mycoplasmas. *Int. J. Syst. Evol. Bacteriol.* **1974**, *24*, 160–171. [CrossRef]
22. Gautier-Bouchardon, A.V. Antimicrobial resistance in mycoplasma spp. *Microbiol. Spectr.* **2018**, *6*. [CrossRef]
23. Hannan, P.C. Guidelines and recommendations for antimicrobial minimum inhibitory concentration (MIC) testing against veterinary mycoplasma species. International research programme on comparative mycoplasmology. *Vet. Res.* **2000**, *31*, 373–395. [CrossRef] [PubMed]
24. Lysnyansky, I.; Ayling, R.D. Mycoplasma bovis: Mechanisms of resistance and trends in antimicrobial susceptibility. *Front. Microbiol.* **2016**, *7*. [CrossRef] [PubMed]
25. Arcangioli, M.-A.; Duet, A.; Meyer, G.; Dernburg, A.; Bézille, P.; Poumarat, F.; Le Grand, D. The role of *Mycoplasma bovis* in bovine respiratory disease outbreaks in veal calf feedlots. *Vet. J.* **2008**, *177*, 89–93. [CrossRef]
26. Nicholas, R.A.J. Bovine mycoplasmosis: Silent and deadly. *Vet. Rec.* **2011**, *168*, 459–462. [CrossRef]
27. Radaelli, E.; Luini, M.; Loria, G.R.; Nicholas, R.A.J.; Scanziani, E. Bacteriological, serological, pathological and immunohistochemical studies of *Mycoplasma bovis* respiratory infection in veal calves and adult cattle at slaughter. *Res. Vet. Sci.* **2008**, *85*, 282–290. [CrossRef]
28. Caswell, J.L.; Bateman, K.G.; Cai, H.Y.; Castillo-Alcala, F. *Mycoplasma bovis* in respiratory disease of feedlot cattle. *Vet. Clin. North Am. Food Anim. Pract.* **2010**, *26*, 365–379. [CrossRef]
29. Nielsen, P.K.; Petersen, M.B.; Nielsen, L.R.; Halasa, T.; Toft, N. Latent class analysis of bulk tank milk PCR and ELISA testing for herd level diagnosis of *Mycoplasma bovis*. *Prev. Vet. Med.* **2015**, *121*, 338–342. [CrossRef]
30. Spergser, J.; Macher, K.; Kargl, M.; Lysnyansky, I.; Rosengarten, R. Emergence, re-emergence, spread and host species crossing of *Mycoplasma bovis* in the Austrian Alps caused by a single endemic strain. *Vet. Microbiol.* **2013**, *164*, 299–306. [CrossRef]
31. Van Engelen, E.; Dijkman, R.; Holzhauer, M.; Junker, K.; Van Wuyckhuise, L.; Gonggrijp, M. Typing of *Mycoplasma bovis* from arthritis outbreaks in dairy herds. In Proceedings of the European Mycoplasma Meeting: Progress in Human and Animal Mycoplasmology, Pendik, Istanbul, Turkey, 3–5 June 2015.
32. Aebi, M.; van den Borne, B.H.P.; Raemy, A.; Steiner, A.; Pilo, P.; Bodmer, M. *Mycoplasma bovis* infections in Swiss dairy cattle: A clinical investigation. *Acta Vet. Scand.* **2015**, *57*, 10. [CrossRef] [PubMed]
33. Arcangioli, M.A.; Chazel, M.; Sellal, E.; Botrel, M.A.; Bezille, P.; Poumarat, F.; Calavas, D.; Le Grand, D. Prevalence of *Mycoplasma bovis* udder infection in dairy cattle: Preliminary field investigation in southeast France. *N. Z. Vet. J.* **2011**, *59*, 75–78. [CrossRef] [PubMed]
34. Filioussis, G.; Christodoulopoulos, G.; Thatcher, A.; Petridou, V.; Bourtzi-Chatzopoulou, E. Isolation of *Mycoplasma bovis* from bovine clinical mastitis cases in Northern Greece. *Vet. J.* **2007**, *173*, 215–218. [CrossRef] [PubMed]
35. Nicholas, R.A.J.; Fox, L.K.; Lysnyansky, I. Mycoplasma mastitis in cattle: To cull or not to cull. *Vet. J.* **2016**, *216*, 142–147. [CrossRef] [PubMed]
36. Passchyn, P.; Piepers, S.; De Meulemeester, L.; Boyen, F.; Haesebrouck, F.; De Vliegher, S. Between-herd prevalence of *Mycoplasma bovis* in bulk milk in Flanders, Belgium. *Res. Vet. Sci.* **2012**, *92*, 219–220. [CrossRef]
37. Klein, U.; de Jong, A.; Moyaert, H.; El Garch, F.; Leon, R.; Richard-Mazet, A.; Rose, M.; Maes, D.; Pridmore, A.; Thomson, J.R.; et al. Antimicrobial susceptibility monitoring of Mycoplasma hyopneumoniae and *Mycoplasma bovis* isolated in Europe. *Vet. Microbiol.* **2017**, *204*, 188–193. [CrossRef]
38. Klein, U.; de Jong, A.; Youala, M.; El Garch, F.; Stevenin, C.; Moyaert, H.; Rose, M.; Catania, S.; Gyuranecz, M.; Pridmore, A.; et al. New antimicrobial susceptibility data from monitoring of *Mycoplasma bovis* isolated in Europe. *Vet. Microbiol.* **2019**, *238*, 108432. [CrossRef]
39. Ministerio de Agricultura, Pesca y Alimentación. Available online: https://www.mapa.gob.es/ (accessed on 20 April 2020).
40. Haapala, V.; Pohjanvirta, T.; Vähänikkilä, N.; Halkilahti, J.; Simonen, H.; Pelkonen, S.; Soveri, T.; Simojoki, H.; Autio, T. Semen as a source of *Mycoplasma bovis* mastitis in dairy herds. *Vet. Microbiol.* **2018**, *216*, 60–66. [CrossRef]
41. Becker, C.A.M.; Thibault, F.M.; Arcangioli, M.-A.; Tardy, F. Loss of diversity within *Mycoplasma bovis* isolates collected in France from bovines with respiratory diseases over the last 35 years. *Infect. Genet. Evol.* **2015**, *33*, 118–126. [CrossRef]

42. Khalil, D.; Becker, C.A.M.; Tardy, F. Alterations in the quinolone resistance-determining regions and fluoroquinolone resistance in clinical isolates and laboratory-derived Mutants of *Mycoplasma bovis*: Not all genotypes may be equal. *Appl. Environ. Microbiol.* **2016**, *82*, 1060–1068. [CrossRef]
43. Khalil, D.; Becker, C.A.M.; Tardy, F. Monitoring the decrease in susceptibility to ribosomal RNAs targeting antimicrobials and its molecular basis in clinical *Mycoplasma bovis* isolates over time. *Microb. Drug Resist. Larchmt. N* **2017**, *23*, 799–811. [CrossRef] [PubMed]
44. Lysnyansky, I.; Mikula, I.; Gerchman, I.; Levisohn, S. Rapid detection of a point mutation in the parC gene associated with decreased susceptibility to fluoroquinolones in *Mycoplasma bovis*. *Antimicrob. Agents Chemother.* **2009**, *53*, 4911–4914. [CrossRef] [PubMed]
45. Mustafa, R.; Qi, J.; Ba, X.; Chen, Y.; Hu, C.; Liu, X.; Tu, L.; Peng, Q.; Chen, H.; Guo, A. In vitro quinolones susceptibility analysis of Chinese *Mycoplasma bovis* isolates and their phylogenetic scenarios based upon QRDRs of DNA topoisomerases revealing a unique transition in ParC. *Pak. Vet. J.* **2013**, *33*, 364–369.
46. Sato, T.; Okubo, T.; Usui, M.; Higuchi, H.; Tamura, Y. Amino acid substitutions in GyrA and ParC are associated with fluoroquinolone resistance in *Mycoplasma bovis* isolates from Japanese dairy calves. *J. Vet. Med. Sci.* **2013**, *75*, 1063–1065. [CrossRef]
47. Sulyok, K.M.; Kreizinger, Z.; Wehmann, E.; Lysnyansky, I.; Bányai, K.; Marton, S.; Jerzsele, Á.; Rónai, Z.; Turcsányi, I.; Makrai, L.; et al. Mutations associated with decreased susceptibility to seven antimicrobial families in field and laboratory-derived *Mycoplasma bovis* strains. *Antimicrob. Agents Chemother.* **2017**, *61*. [CrossRef]
48. Hata, E.; Harada, T.; Itoh, M. Relationship between antimicrobial susceptibility and multilocus sequence type of *Mycoplasma bovis* isolates and development of a method for rapid detection of point mutations involved in decreased susceptibility to macrolides, lincosamides, tetracyclines, and spectinomycin. *Appl. Environ. Microbiol.* **2019**, *85*. [CrossRef]
49. Lerner, U.; Amram, E.; Ayling, R.D.; Mikula, I.; Gerchman, I.; Harrus, S.; Teff, D.; Yogev, D.; Lysnyansky, I. Acquired resistance to the 16-membered macrolides tylosin and tilmicosin by *Mycoplasma bovis*. *Vet. Microbiol.* **2014**, *168*, 365–371. [CrossRef]
50. Lysnyansky, I.; Gerchman, I.; Flaminio, B.; Catania, S. Decreased susceptibility to macrolide-lincosamide in mycoplasma synoviae is associated with mutations in 23S ribosomal RNA. *Microb. Drug Resist.* **2015**, *21*, 581–589. [CrossRef]
51. Amram, E.; Mikula, I.; Schnee, C.; Ayling, R.D.; Nicholas, R.A.J.; Rosales, R.S.; Harrus, S.; Lysnyansky, I. 16S rRNA gene mutations associated with decreased susceptibility to tetracycline in *Mycoplasma bovis*. *Antimicrob. Agents Chemother.* **2015**, *59*, 796–802. [CrossRef]
52. CIMAVet. Centro de Información de Medicamentos para Veterinaria. Available online: https://cimavet.aemps.es/ (accessed on 20 April 2020).
53. Stipkovits, L.; Ripley, P.H.; Tenk, M.; Glávits, R.; Molnár, T.; Fodor, L. The efficacy of valnemulin (Econor) in the control of disease caused by experimental infection of calves with *Mycoplasma bovis*. *Res. Vet. Sci.* **2005**, *78*, 207–215. [CrossRef]
54. Waites, K.B.; Bébéar, C.M.; Robertson, J.A.; Talkington, D.F.; Kenny, G.E. *Cumitech 34: Laboratory Diagnosis of Mycoplasmal Infections*; American Society for Microbiology: Washington, WA, USA, 2001.
55. Tola, S.; Angioi, A.; Rocchigiani, A.M.; Idini, G.; Manunta, D.; Galleri, G.; Leori, G. Detection of *Mycoplasma agalactiae* in sheep milk samples by polymerase chain reaction. *Vet. Microbiol.* **1997**, *54*, 17–22. [CrossRef]
56. Foddai, A.; Idini, G.; Fusco, M.; Rosa, N.; De la Fe, C.; Zinellu, S.; Corona, L.; Tola, S. Rapid differential diagnosis of *Mycoplasma agalactiae* and *Mycoplasma bovis* based on a multiplex-PCR and a PCR-RFLP. *Mol. Cell. Probes* **2005**, *19*, 207–212. [CrossRef] [PubMed]
57. Tamura, K.; Stecher, G.; Peterson, D.; Filipski, A.; Kumar, S. MEGA6: Molecular evolutionary genetics analysis version 6.0. *Mol. Biol. Evol.* **2013**, *30*, 2725–2729. [CrossRef] [PubMed]
58. Gómez-Martín, A.; De la Fe, C.; Amores, J.; Sánchez, A.; Contreras, A.; Paterna, A.; Buendía, A.J.; Corrales, J.C. Anatomic location of *Mycoplasma mycoides* subsp. *capri* and *Mycoplasma agalactiae* in naturally infected goat male auricular carriers. *Vet. Microbiol.* **2012**, *157*, 355–362. [CrossRef]
59. Albers, A.C.; Fletcher, R.D. Simple method for quantitation of viable mycoplasmas. *Appl. Environ. Microbiol.* **1982**, *43*, 958–960. [CrossRef] [PubMed]
60. Epi Info^{TM}|CDC. Available online: https://www.cdc.gov/epiinfo/index.html (accessed on 20 April 2020).

61. Babraham Bioinformatics—FastQC A Quality Control Tool for High Throughput Sequence Data. Available online: https://www.bioinformatics.babraham.ac.uk/projects/fastqc/ (accessed on 20 April 2020).
62. Li, H.; Durbin, R. Fast and accurate short read alignment with Burrows-Wheeler transform. *Bioinformatics* **2009**, *25*, 1754–1760. [CrossRef]
63. Okonechnikov, K.; Conesa, A.; García-Alcalde, F. Qualimap 2: Advanced multi-sample quality control for high-throughput sequencing data. *Bioinformatics* **2016**, *32*, 292–294. [CrossRef]
64. Thorvaldsdóttir, H.; Robinson, J.T.; Mesirov, J.P. Integrative Genomics Viewer (IGV): High-performance genomics data visualization and exploration. *Brief. Bioinform.* **2013**, *14*, 178–192. [CrossRef]
65. Deatherage, D.E.; Barrick, J.E. Identification of mutations in laboratory-evolved microbes from next-generation sequencing data using breseq. In *Engineering and Analyzing Multicellular Systems*; Humana Press: New York, NY, USA, 2014; Volume 1151, pp. 165–188. [CrossRef]

MDPI
St. Alban-Anlage 66
4052 Basel
Switzerland
Tel. +41 61 683 77 34
Fax +41 61 302 89 18
www.mdpi.com

Pathogens Editorial Office
E-mail: pathogens@mdpi.com
www.mdpi.com/journal/pathogens

www.ingramcontent.com/pod-product-compliance
Lightning Source LLC
LaVergne TN
LVHW070613100526
838202LV00012B/635